Praise For

In the Garden: A 40-Day Journey of Hope and Healing

In the Garden: A 40-day Journey of Hope and Healing is more than a journey of food and faith. It is a journey of heart, passion, and promise. Author, Nichole Fogleman, shares her knowledge on healthy eating along with her love for the Lord, her knowledge of Scripture, and her authentic heart. Taking the journey through this book is going on a journey with a knowledgeable guide, an encouraging friend, and a woman guided by the Holy Spirit to reflect her love for helping and loving others in our world. Along this journey, you learn from relatable real-life stories from the author as well as healthy life-giving food habits that are conveyed in a language that allows the reader to lose intimidation and with confidence believe this new method of plant-based living is attainable. This book is love-giving and life-changing!

—Rev Abbie D. Duenckel
Author of the weekly blog www.luke8women.com

Last winter I was personally going through aggressive chemotherapies, and I implemented some of Nichole and her husband's advice written in this book. I immediately noticed a difference, more energy, better mood, no bloated stomach, and nervous bowels. Thank God now I am in remission. Pet scan and two blood checkups are all clear. Prayers, eating style, and medicine are all we can do from our side. The rest is up to our sovereign God. And I had a special peace knowing that I'm doing everything that is on my side and knowing that God has a perfect plan for the outcome.

I have been in Christian ministry for 12 years currently working as a missionary for Cru International in Macedonia. I've never put a lot of focus on what the Bible has to say about eating plants, seeds, olives, figs, other vegetables, and fruits etc. I'm amazed at how much the Bible has to say about it. I'm so grateful that Nichole put her long years of personal experience and scientific research into a book. Her writing style is noticeably clear, practical, sincere, personal, and humble. It's easy for the reader to connect with her. Once I read the book "Purpose Driven Life" and undertook the 40 days to complete the book and it impacted my life a lot. I believe the same is true for this 40-day journey of ***In the Garden: a 40-day Journey of Hope and Healing***.

—**Zlatko Buchkoski**, Christian minister, and author of the book, "God's Fingerprints" (English title) Sharing the gospel in every pore of society. Influencing the young lost generation with Christian values. Educator. Digital strategist & social media activist *Christ is the sole solution for soul pollution*

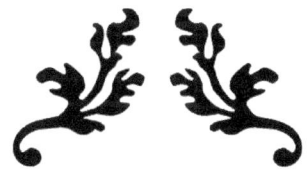

IN THE GARDEN

A 40-Day Journey of Hope and Healing

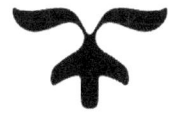

Nichole Fogleman

Published by KHARIS PUBLISHING, an imprint of
KHARIS MEDIA LLC.
Copyright © 2022 Nichole Fogleman
ISBN-13: 978-1-63746-174-7
ISBN-10: 1-63746-174-7

Library of Congress Control Number: 2022945973

All rights reserved. This book or parts thereof may not be reproduced in any form, stored in a retrieval system, or transmitted in any form by any means - electronic, mechanical, photocopy, recording, or otherwise - without prior written permission of the publisher, except as provided by United States of America copyright law.

Scripture taken from THE HOLY BIBLE, ENGLISH STANDARD VERSION ® Copyright© 2001 by Crossway, a publishing ministry of Good News Publishers. Used by permission.

All KHARIS PUBLISHING products are available at special quantity discounts for bulk purchase for sales promotions, premiums, fund-raising, and educational needs. For details, contact:

Kharis Media LLC
Tel: 1-479-599-8657
support@kharispublishing.com
www.kharispublishing.com

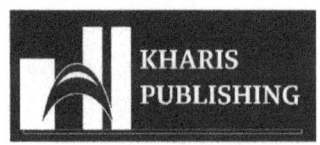

This book is dedicated to my mom, Lynda "D"
You were a complete work of beauty inside and out

Introduction

Welcome to a journey. A journey to take you to a new level of living. This is not a self-help book, diet book, or cookbook. It's a book to share the secrets I have discovered on how to live a better life with two essential ingredients: food and faith. Throughout the pages of this book, I will share with you science-based resources for healing with food, a study of God's Word to accompany your journey, and hope.

This book is about immersing yourself in plant-based eating and the study of God's Word for 40 days. A 40-day challenge. The significance of 40 in the Bible is undeniable. Christian author, Nicki Koziarz defines this significance with, "the number forty signifies new life, growth, transformation, and change. But it can also represent a time of trial, testing, or judgment." I can guarantee all of these elements during these 40 days, but the hope is that you will receive life-changing healing and never look back on your former life.

Who am I as the writer of this challenge? By profession, I am a nurse that specializes in pain. I'm the one that guides you to the operating room, gently speaks calming words as you inhale the fresh air, then drifts you off to sleep, and of course, takes care of your vital organs while you enjoy your slumber. Through the years, understanding the why, how, and when of pain has filled my life. Learning about pain has been a personal mission. My mom struggled with severe chronic pain impacting her life and our family for 20 years. I have experienced my struggles with pain while recovering from a double mastectomy and ankle reconstruction. At work, I meet people daily that struggle with pain. And unfortunately, we live in a world where the control of pain has turned many lives upside down, with addiction, sickness, and death. The mission God has placed upon me is to help you with your struggle either big or small. I am honored to help.

This book ended up being much more than just a devotional. I poured out on these pages stories about my journey with generational sin. When the writing process began, this was not the intention, but God always has bigger plans. Writing about scripture and discovering mysteries in God's Word is one of my passions. "In the Garden" began as a collection of scriptures interwoven about food and agriculture in the Bible. Then God started to whisper Deuteronomy 8:8 in my ear, and somehow the book took a life of its own. Deuteronomy 8:7 begins with the promise from God that "He is bringing you into a good land" and that is the goal of this book. He wants to bring you into a good land of hope and healing.

Why did I choose a plant-based lifestyle? This journey began little by little 15 years ago when our youngest daughter was diagnosed with Attention Deficit Hyperactivity Disorder (ADHD). Instead of reaching for Ritalin, we reached for scientific journals and research. We completely restructured our diets, and things began to change. We saw the power of food in detoxifying the body. Our youngest daughter's ability to focus changed dramatically and 10 years after, she was accepted into one of the top high school programs in our state based on her writing and reading skills.

As our journey with food continued, we learned more and more. At some point, my husband came across the story of Dr. Max Gerson and his cure rate of cancer with juicing. At the age of 29, I was diagnosed with melanoma, and this became the forefront of my husband's mind to keep his loved ones free of diseases and illness. Being a scientist, he saw what food did for his daughter, and the search for answers only became stronger. Thankfully, the search became easier with the production of amazing documentaries like *Fat, Sick and nearly Dead and Super-Size Me*, introducing us to a plethora of physicians and scientists in the plant-based community. Then *The China Study* was published by Colin Campbell, and we were sold. We have been eating mostly plants now for ten years. Do we ever cheat? Sure, we do. Giving up cheese was the most difficult process. The journey became more about cultivation, reaping rewards little by little. We have seen rewards. We are both in our fifties, we rarely get sick, our blood work is impeccable, our doctor's checkups indicate freedom of disease, we run for exercise, we hike, and pretty much do any activity we choose and feel great doing it.

Then I read the book by Neal Bernard, *Foods that Fight Pain*, and discovered that diet could be an answer to heal the body and free individuals from pain. After recovering from major surgery from a foot injury, I instituted Bernard's food fighting techniques on myself and realized they worked. I immersed myself in the study of inflammation and fighting free radicals to reverse the consequences of toxins placed in our bodies.

This same year, my mom began eating plant-based, not 100%, more like 60%. She suffered from arachnoiditis from an iatrogenic injury in her 30s. She incorporated the lifestyle slowly. On Sundays, we took turns creating recipes together for fun. Her pain improved significantly while she was eating more plants. Unfortunately, her last moments on earth were complicated by a failing pain pump and the Delta Covid epidemic; she went to be with her savior in Heaven, in the fall of 2021.

These pages have taught me so many things, so many things that I need to work on, and so many things that I still do not know or understand. The Word of God is a living thing that teaches new lessons and shows new mysteries every time you dig deep. In my practice, I try to spend forty days every year studying the Word in a straight sequence. Doing this practice will change your life. You will come out of this a different person. This person that reemerges may not be recognizable to friends and family. And with this comes different vices, because you will realize that you are no longer of this world, you are just living "in" this world.

Thank you for allowing me the honor to write this study for those that live in persistent pain. Thank you for allowing me the honor to write this study for those that struggle with chronic illness. Thank you to my husband for allowing me to write these words, the ups and downs that it brings when completely immersed in a task. Thank you, Dear precious Heavenly Father, Holy One, righteous above all others, for allowing me to spend these days with you and writing your words. I am forever grateful to be your child.

The format of this book goes as follows: there are six chapters, and each chapter has six days to immerse yourself in scripture. On the seventh day of each week, we rest. Each week, we will place ourselves in the gardens that are sprinkled throughout scripture, from the land of Eden to the promised land of the Israelites, to the prophets of old, and the gardens and terrain in Jesus' days. Many of the references to gardens will be metaphorical comparing our souls and bodies to the seeds, fruits, and trees of the ancient Holy Land. And then splattered throughout the book will be practical advice about eating a plant-based diet and incorporating this lifestyle into your daily habits. Each day along with the scripture study will be daily tips to get you through the forty days. The scriptures quoted are from the ESV version of the bible unless specified otherwise.

Welcome to this journey, 40 days to a new you!
Nichole

   Welcome to the Hope for Pain Journey, where we immerse ourselves in God's Word and plants for 40 days. We will eat plants together, learn lessons from the bible, and heal our bodies together as a community. Each chapter will be filled with resources, personal stories, recommendations for eating a plant-based diet, recipes, and immersing you in God's holy Word. The Hope for Pain dietary plan is your resource for powering your body with plants for 40 days.

   The word "vegan will not be use." I feel it adds extra stress and anxiety to the concept of eating plant-based. I also want to avoid the stereotypes that come with the word. Instead, I will try to focus on eating local, sustainable foods that live in either a garden or in the produce aisle. I also believe it is important to incorporate plant-based eating as a lifestyle rather than a diet. Many people try different diets and then give up because they find themselves craving/bingeing restricted foods. Instead of treating plant-based eating as a fad diet, treat it like a lifestyle. The lifestyle approach is the reason we promote the 80% plant-based plan. Each day, we will explore in more details the elements of this plan.

   I have created a go-to guide for switching to a plant-based lifestyle. The guide details specific substitutes for items you may be eating currently that you need to remove for the next 40 days. Remember that if you make a mistake or have a cheat day, you can always return to the roots of this lifestyle. I encourage you to take your produce aisle by storm or discover your green thumb in a fresh outdoor garden.

   Not only is it important to adopt a plant-based lifestyle, it is also key to make sure the plants and produce you are eating are fresh, organic, or local (if possible). This is a healing journey. Sometimes prepackaged items contain extra ingredients that don't fall into your new diet/lifestyle. If you read the back of the packaging and find that you don't know some of the ingredients, try to steer clear. The goal is to eat as many raw foods as possible, with the fewest ingredients.

The Plan

Remove these…
Beverages: alcohol, coffee, caffeinated teas, carbonated beverages, all artificial sweeteners

Replace with these…
Beverages: freshly extracted vegetable juices, distilled water, caffeine-free herbal teas

Remove these…
Dairy: all milk, cheese, ice cream, whipped toppings, and non-dairy creamers

Replace with these…
Dairy: fresh almond milk, non-dairy cheese, rice milk, coconut milk, soymilk, oat milk

Remove these…
Fruits: canned and sweetened fruits, along with non-organic and sulfured dried fruits

Replace with these…
Fruits: all fresh organic, as well as unsulfured organic dried fruits

Remove these…
Refined and or enriched grains: refined, bleached flour products, most cold breakfast cereals, and white rice

Replace with these...
Whole-grain cereals, bread, pasta, brown rice, soaked oats, raw muesli, dehydrated granola

Remove These ...
Meat: beef, pork, fish, chicken, eggs, turkey, hamburgers, hot dogs, bacon, sausage, bologna

Replace with these...
Meat substitutes: all cooked beans, mushrooms, sprouted beans, chia seeds, wheatgrass

Remove these...
All roasted and or salted nuts and seeds

Replace with these...
Sunflower seeds, macadamia nuts, walnuts, raw almond butter, tahini, cashews, and almonds

Remove these...
Oils: all lard, margarine, shortenings, and anything containing hydrogenated oils or trans fats

Replace with these...
Oils and fats: extra virgin olive oil (sparingly), flaxseed oil, avocados,

Remove these...
Sweets: all refined white or brown sugar, sugar syrups, chocolate, candy, gum, cookies, donuts, cakes, pies

Replace with these...
Sweets: fruit smoothies, raw unfiltered honey, stevia, agave nectar, pure maple syrup, carob

Remove these...
Seasonings: refined table salt and any seasoning containing it.

Replace with these...
Seasonings: fresh or dehydrated herbs, garlic, sweet onions, parsley, salt-free seasonings, unrefined sea salt (sparingly)

Build houses and live in them, and plant gardens and eat their produce.
—*Jeremiah 29:5*

Table of Contents

FIGS
- Day 1: 20
- Day 2: 23
- Day 3: 25
- Day 4: 29
- Day 5: 32
- Day 6: 34
- Day 7: 37

SEEDS
- Day 8: 40
- Day 9: 43
- Day 10: 46
- Day 11: 49
- Day 12: 52
- Day 13: 55
- Day 14: 57

THE FORMER AND LATTER RAIN
- Day 15: 60
- Day 16: 64
- Day 17: 67
- Day 18: 70
- Day 19: 72

Day 20: 75
Day 21: 77

THE FRUIT OF THE SPIRIT

Day 22: 80
Day 23: 82
Day 24: 85
Day 25: 87
Day 26: 90
Day 27: 93
Day 28: 95

THE FRUIT OF THE VINE

Day 29: 100
Day 30: 102
Day 31: 105
Day 32: 107
Day 33: 110
Day 34: 112
Day 35: 114

THE OLIVE TREE

Day 36: 118
Day 37: 121
Day 38: 124
Day 39: 127
Day 40: 130
About Kharis Publishing *136*
Cited reference *137*

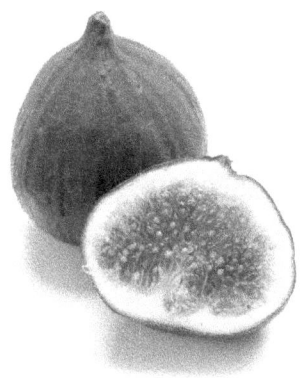

FIGS

Day 1:

Scripture Reading: Genesis 2:5-9

And out of the ground the Lord God made to spring up every tree that is pleasant to the sight and good for food. Genesis 2:9

Have you ever noticed how often God's Word speaks about trees, gardens, land, soil, wheat, vineyards, and food? God's Word contains secrets within its text, and we are called to explore the mysteries hidden there, the mystery about the healing nature of God's creation. God wants us to sift through His Word and discover His mysteries. In this chapter, we will explore the mystery of the fig tree, the queen of all trees. She is mentioned often in the scripture. She lives in a symbiotic relationship with her creator and exists only by relationship.

Trees encircle many of my earliest memories. I grew up in the deep south where fruit trees were grown in every plot of land, taking my consciousness to a place with a house, a lake, cows, gardens, and many fruit trees. This plot of land was where my life began. It was this land that brought me to God. Trees to the left, trees to the right, flowering trees, and those with the juiciest fruit imaginable. In the front yard lies the fig tree. As a child, I never paid that much attention to this tree. But as an adult, visiting grandparents, I stood under the leaves of the tree, admiring the abundance of fruit, and realized that I had experienced a gift like no other. I had lived in Eden. The beauty, the sweetness, and the sin. I learned who God was in that Eden. He began to reveal himself to me on that soil under the shelter of those trees. I learned about sin, violence, anger, fear, and sexual temptations in this place. I pause under the fig tree now to understand its fruit, and its meaning, to share my story, to share the things I have learned journeying this earth

Do you have a place in your memory that takes you back in time? Can you see this place? Anxiety can creep in as we begin a new journey. Doubt and distractions may squirm their way into your thoughts. Close your eyes, take a moment, find a quiet place, and find that memory that brings you peace. My place is the lake on that land: swimming, frolicking, fishing. Throughout this journey, the place that you find hidden in your memories will be very important. You will go there when you are feeling anxious or restless. You have only one goal on this first day, finding your place and spending some time alone in your place (figuratively or literally), imagining what life could look like after a journey of 40 days.

Today's Tip: Each day I will share a practical tip about adopting a plant-based lifestyle for the next 40 days.

"If it came from a plant, eat it; if it was made in a plant, don't." (Michael Pollan, author of the Omnivore's Dilemma). (1)

In the Garden

That sentence pretty much sums it up. The goal during the forty days is to eat plants and heal your body. We are going to avoid all processed foods. Unfortunately, commercial companies try to monopolize food trends. There are a lot of yummy-tasting products that are being produced that appear to be "plant-based." Even Burger King makes their version of the plant-based burger using the "Beyond Burger." Don't fall for the trap. These are not good for you. For the next forty days try to only eat items that have less than six ingredients on the ingredient label, the less the better. Each day will get easier and easier. Fill your pantry with fruits and vegetables, seeds, and grains. Review the dietary plan on page 1.

Day 2:

Scripture reading for the day: Amos 1:1, Amos 7: 14-15

I was no prophet, nor a prophet's son, but I was a herdsman and a dresser of sycamore figs. Amos 7:14

The man was Amos. He took care of sycamore-fig trees. It was no small consequence that Amos cared for fig trees. God never mentions things in His word without some type of meaning. They are essential to his story and his purpose.

Amos was just a man when he was called by God. He was called by God because of his vocation and his proximity. He lived only 12 miles south of the border. Not the border you imagine today, but a border that existed thousands of years ago between two kingdoms. Israel in the north and Judah in the south. Jesus was from the same southern kingdom, Judah. Amos lived there 750 years before Jesus walked the earth. Amos cultivated and cared for God's creation. He became a messenger, a person called by God to proclaim the truth. Spend a little time today outside in nature or look out the window. Find a tree and observe its beauty. Observe the creatures that enjoy the trees. And then think about this young man, Amos. Think about how you would feel if God called you; Amos, just tending to his daily routine of life with no agenda or purpose. What would you do?

Tomorrow, we will explore more details about this tree and its symbiotic relationship with its creator. For today you have a simple task, power your body with plants and focus on the beauty of nature that surrounds you. Journal about this experience. Which tree did you

In the Garden

choose? Which creatures did you see? Do you feel a sense of calm and peace when standing or sitting among her branches?

_____

_____

_____

_____

_____

_____

_____

Today's Tips: Go through your pantry and get rid of temptations. Throw away those foods that lead you down the wrong path. We all have them. Salty snacks are my kryptonite. Let your family know that you are on this journey. Invite them to do it with you. It will be much easier if the sweets and salty snacks are removed from the kitchen. Ask your family to hide their snacks so you don't see them.

Day 3:

Scripture Reading: Genesis 3:7, Micah, 4:4, Zechariah 3:10

Every one of you will invite his neighbor to come under his vine and under his fig tree saith the Lord of Hosts. Zechariah 3:10

The fig tree existed on the earth from the very beginning. She lived in the very first garden; the Garden of Eden. There is something very unique about the fig tree and the way it is pollinated. Her flowers are on the inside of her fruit and are pollinated only by a specific species of wasps, the little tiny fig wasp. The only task this wasp has is to pollinate the flowers within the fig fruit. That is her only purpose, to pollinate the fruit on the fig tree. The fruit cannot ripen without this relationship. The tree is completely dependent on their relationship.

She, the fig tree, was plentiful in this fertile land and still is to this day. References to this tree can be found over and over again in scripture. Even Jesus while speaking about the end times referred to the fig tree. (Matthew 24: 32-36) The fig tree usually bears fruit two to three times per year. In the spring, it is the last to produce leaves signifying that summer is near.

But let's focus on the theme of the symbiotic relationship. Could this be the mystery of this story? Did Amos appreciate the symbiotic relationship between the fig and the wasp? If a fig is not pollinated, then this fruit never ripens. It's considered bad fruit, as Jeremiah remarked in his prophetic word in Jeremiah 24:2-3. Amos witnessed the mutually beneficial relationship between the tree and the wasp and knew that it was essential to bear fruit. His observations may have led him to a greater understanding of the importance of a symbiotic relationship with God, enabling him to fulfill his purpose of speaking prophecy to his neighbors.

Charles Spurgeon, the famous British theologian, and pastor, once spoke about symbiotic relationships in a sermon. I love to read his old sermons. He noted that every past spiritual leader distanced themselves from their followers, there was no relationship, just reverence, and worship. But this was different with Jesus;" he loves having all his followers live near him; he loves to have them in sympathy with him; he loves to make them feel that, while he is their superior and their King, he is also as their fellow, bone of their bone, and flesh of their flesh, ... One object of Christ's religion is, to bring all his disciples into union and communion with its great Founder, that they may have fellowship with the Father, and with his Son, Jesus Christ." (2)

This type of relationship is what God has in mind even today. Jesus said "Abide in Me, and I in you. I am the vine; you *are* the branches. He who abides in Me, and I in him, bears much fruit; for without Me you can do nothing." (John 15:4-5)

Are you ready to have this type of relationship with God? Are you open to having this give-and-take symbiotic relationship? Webster defines this type of relationship as "living in or being a close physical association between two or more dissimilar organisms." There is interdependence. Do you struggle to be dependent on others?

Since I was a little girl, taking fruit from the fruit trees, there was an interdependence I felt with God. I don't know why it happened. I just knew Him. He was there. I never questioned His existence. I came to know Jesus as my savior at a very early age and never questioned his supreme existence in my life. By no means have I lived a perfect life. And most likely the story is different for you. And that is ok. Maybe there's trust issue, a father figure that betrayed you. This same God that called Amos, is reliable. He is the same merciful father that wants to love and know you.

I have to be honest, at this very moment, my mom is dying. I'm sitting with her in the hospital. She has suffered for years with chronic pain. I'll tell you more about her struggles and victories later in the pages of this book. In the last five years of her life, she learned to rely on her Heavenly Father. It was so hard for her. But her last five years were so good. She learned how to let go, and only rely on Him. I sit here now holding her hand, air Pod in my ears listening to the words from the song "I surrender" on repeat. The precious words in my ears, "Here I am, down on my knees again, surrendering all. I know you heed my cries. I want to know you more. More of you, less of me" I surrender. I surrender my mom to you, Lord Jesus.

Today during your Bible study and quiet time think about the relationships in your life. Make some notes. Which relationships do you value most? What makes these relationships valuable? Is it because you truly trust them? Being with them, does it feel so comfortable you never want to leave? Say a silent prayer and thank God today for these relationships in your life.

_____

_____

_____

_____

_____

_____

Today's Tip: Expect detox symptoms. As you cleanse your body of toxins, it is very normal for your body to go through a detox process, possibly as early as the 3rd day. You may experience headaches, nausea, rashes pimples, diarrhea, and constipation. Author of the plant-based

Hallelujah diet, George Malkmus recommends not giving up, stating "I assure you it will pass, and when it does, you'll feel fantastic- better than you may have felt for years!" (3)

Day 4:

Scripture Reading: Amos 7:14-16

I was no prophet, nor a prophet's son, but I was a herdsman, and a dresser of sycamore figs. Amos 7:14

When Amos was called by the Lord, he was the first of the prophets called. Before Isaiah, before Jeremiah. There was no precedent to fashion his ministry. He was a simple man, taking care of his fig trees, a dresser of figs. How in the world does one dress a fig? The word dresser is translated from Hebrew as "boless shikmim" meaning piercer of sycamore figs. The mystery of this custom is beautiful. Today we will focus on the meaning of this word, its significance, and its mystery in the living Word.

The fig tree may have been in the first garden, but after sin entered creation, scientists believed that the sycamore fig tree proliferated the plains of Africa, their seeds once again traveled from the Nile River banks to the desert of Israel. To this day in Africa, for figs to ripen, human hands are required to pierce the figs for the ripening process to take place. (4) The dresser must carefully bruise or gnash each fig on the tree. The ripening process occurs quickly after the gnashing. Most likely Amos was a gifted gnasher, and bruiser, of these precious trees.

Bruising. Does your story, and your journey here on earth involve any type of bruising? At worse, is physical abuse part of your story? Do you experience triggering events from your past bruises? Remember the place I told you about on day one, the place I go to in my mind if I need to relax or de-stress? That was the place where I first learned about bruising. I saw some things in that house that one does not forget quickly.

In the Garden

The beautiful and mysterious part of the process of dressing the sycamore figs, the figs on these trees could not ripen until they were bruised. This is true of all sycamore-fig trees in ancient times; a human hand had to bruise them for them to ripen.

My story, the sinful justification behind the bruising that I witnessed was carried over from generation to generation. Not the bruising, but the sin that first caused the hand to lift. However, I would not be writing these words on paper today, experiencing the ripening process, if I had not gone through this unfolding of generational sin that began 55 years ago. I am the person that God created, for the good or the bad, because of those events. God is continually ripening me.

Today spend some time with this beautiful metaphor, bruising to ripening. Begin to write your own story. Afterward, we will together start to connect the dots and witness how God has started ripening your soul. For many of us, this ripening process equates with the process of healing. That is what this journey of 40 days is all about. So, get your pen, don't waste a moment, and write it all out.

_____

_____

_____

_____

_____

_____

_____

_____

Nichole Fogleman

Today's Tip: Start exploring recipes.

At the end of each chapter, I will share one of my favorite "go-to" recipes. I am not a trained cook. I am just like you. I find great recipes on Instagram and in books. The following are my favorite individuals to follow on Instagram. These individuals are very passionate about eating plant-based and sharing their journey. A couple of them may not be 100% vegan but have some great recipes using vegetables. Tomorrow I will share my favorite books. But don't reinvent the wheel. Make it fun and start exploring. If you don't have Instagram, then download it today. If you don't have internet, go to the local library and start googling plant-based recipes.

Instagram favorites: go to the search button, type in these names, and follow these individuals:

> vegetarian vids, Lauren Kretzer, the Nordic kitchen, couple cooks, loving vegan ks, loving it vegan, go plant-strong, well plated, crowded kitchen, sculpted kitchen, the vegan sara, the gut health md, Jane Esselstyn, love and lemons, plant based on a budget, forks over knives, easy vegan4u

Day 5:

Scripture Reading: Luke 13:6-9

Sir, let it alone this year also until I dig around it and put on manure.
Luke 13:8

We meet another dresser of the sycamore fig, this one unnamed and possibly fictional, but the author of the parable is no doubt unequal. Yesterday we talked about the need for figs to be handled, bruised by man to ripen. In this story, the trees were not bearing fruit. Jesus told them that "until the vinedresser digs around and adds manure" the figs would not ripen. The King James version uses the word "dung" instead of manure. Gardeners, old and new use manure for fertilizer, but in this case, Jesus was the fertilizer.

After spending a year studying the relationship between the fig and its tree, I discovered an article written by a scientist on the topic of botany. (5) Mysteriously somewhere along the line of history, the figs in Israel no longer required scathing. The figs no longer needed human help to ripen. The trees in Israel have now been metaphorically fertilized by Jesus when he walked the earth, ate from the trees, and sat among their branches.

The same miracle that happened to these trees can happen to us. As Paul said to the Corinthians (2 Corinthians 4:8-10), "We may be hard pressed on every side, but not crushed; perplexed, but not in despair, persecuted but not abandoned, struck down, but not destroyed. We always carry around in our body the death of Jesus so that the life of Jesus may also be revealed in our body." The figs in Israel no longer need bruising and through the power of Jesus Christ, we no longer are crushed, left in despair, or abandoned.

Nichole Fogleman

This ripening process is available for all. If you have never received this miracle of ripening; a ripening that no longer requires the hands of man but is made fully mature by the power of Christ, then I invite you right now where you are, position yourself to your knees if you are able, or just close your eyes, and say this prayer to your Creator. Thank you, Lord, for creating me, for loving me, for forgiving me of my sins, and sending your son, Jesus, to take the bruising, the scathing, the gnashing for my sins, dying on the cross, and rising again, and sitting at the right hand of your throne so now I can have a personal relationship with you while I live here on this earth.

Today's Tip: Cookbooks
Check out your local library or purchase a couple of the following books. These physicians, scientists, registered dieticians, and chefs have done all the hard work for you. The following are some of my favorites. (I have no affiliation with any of these authors or organizations. I just think they are fabulous!)

Plant Based on a Budget by Toni Okamoto; *The Fiber Fueled Cookbook* by Will Bulsiewicz; *Forks over Knives the Cookbook* by Del Sroufe; *The Engine 2 Cookbook* by Rip Esselstyn; *The China Study Cookbook* by Leanne Campbell

Day 6:

Scripture Reading: Isaiah 61: 1-3, Mark 11:12-14, Amos 7:14-15

He has sent me to bind up the brokenhearted, to proclaim freedom for the captives. Isaiah 61:1

Today I want you to place yourself in one or two categories: rich or poor. How do you define rich? Are you rich enough not to worry about placing food on the table next week or gas in the car? Unfortunately, life tends to categorize us into rich or poor. Jesus was born poor. Those that face chronic illness often struggle with finances and live life paycheck to paycheck. And Amos, the young man playing front and center of our study this week was poor.

Most ancient farmers of sycamore fig trees lived by humble means. (5) They were poor, and their fruits were eaten by the poor. Interestingly, Jesus was noted to eat this sacred fruit from its branches on several occasions. Amos's resume was lacking, with no formal education, not related to other prophets or royalty. He worked two jobs and lived in the desert. He was called to speak to the rich, the same individuals that lived recklessly and oppressed his neighbors because of socioeconomic hierarchy. Imagine this occurring today. Imagine a man born in the Appalachian Mountains of West Virginia called to preach to the businessmen of Manhattan, New York, and worse of all he is called to point out their reckless and corrupt lifestyles. So heed this warning, the state of your bank account right now has no bearing on whether God wants to use you for His purposes.

God feels compassion for the poor. Jesus empathizes with the poor. Our scripture reading today from Isaiah, emphasizes that God's spirit wants to proclaim the good news to the poor. The same message spoken by the prophets still applies to us today. Rewrite the words of Isaiah and personalize them. Take the word "them" and place your name. Take the word "poor" and place your name. Place your name in front of the word brokenhearted and captives.

_____

_____

_____

_____

_____

Today's Tip: Eating plant Based on a Budget.
I heard a lot of complaints over the years about eating plants based on a low-income or disability check. Fruits and Vegetables can be expensive, especially if eating organic and out of season. Here are some tips.
1. Eat locally and in season. I have done some of my research in this area. Our local Walmart carries local farmers' produce along with many other chain grocery stores. Aldi's carries fruits and vegetables.
2. Buy frozen vegetables. Many vegetables when frozen are quickly frozen soon after being picked to keep their freshness. This method retains their vitamins and minerals.
3. I've also done some exploring at the dollar store. Our local dollar store carries plant-based milk like soy in cartons, frozen vegetables, and salt-free nuts. Avoid canned vegetables. They

In the Garden

are usually laden with salt but sometimes store brands have less sodium.
4. Eat simply. Potatoes are a simple great whole food, with 11% protein and 0 fat. They are high in Vitamin C, B6, Iron, and Magnesium.
5. Start a garden. I read a statistic recently about how just planting a small garden can produce 300 lbs. of produce worth $600 a year with a $70 investment (6). Seeds are very cheap. You are not going to reap the benefits in 40 days from a garden, but this plan is a process to strive for a healthier lifestyle for the long haul. Do a trade with your neighbor for fresh produce from their garden in exchange for watching their cats. Get creative
.

Day 7:

It's your day of rest. Every seven days we will take a complete day of rest for your body, mind, and soul. The day may fall on a Sunday, Saturday, or Monday. It all just depends on when you started the journey. Today is your day to rest. Enjoy your day off and see you tomorrow.

_____

_____

_____

_____

_____

Black Beans in the Crock-Pot

There is an art to preparing beans and incorporating beans into your diet is pretty much essential to being successful in following this plan. There are two key elements to avoiding the "gassy" feeling when eating beans. Run water over the dry beans to remove any sediment and keep eating them. Your gut will get used to them and your body will eventually thank you. I have found the easiest and most successful way to cook dry beans is in the crock pot. I have tried every possible way known to man. This recipe is the easiest I have found. Use this recommendation to make any dry beans except lentils.

Prepare these early in the week so you can have them on other days.

Ingredients:

1. 1 package of black beans

2. Sea salt

Take the beans and place them in a strainer and run them under water to remove debris. Place beans in crock-pot and cover with water, about 1 inch of water covering. Cook on a 6-hour high setting. If you are gone for the day at work, allow the crock pot to keep the beans warm after the 6-hour cycle is complete. After the beans is done, then add the salt and grab a spoon to taste as you add.

For the meal, prepare brown rice according to the package. In our family when the kids were little, to make a game of this meal, we would ask each child, "Beans over rice or rice over beans?" We still do this today when the kids are home. You decide how you like them. Then add your fixings.

(I'm from the south, and we love the word "fixings" I'm fixing to go get some beans. We are going to add some "fixings" to these beans.)

Fixings

You decide which "fixings" you want to add. Here are some options. No sour cream or cheese!!!

1. Always add a few squirts of lime
2. Salsa from a jar (organic) or make your own to have all week
3. Add some greens - spinach leaves to the top
4. Cilantro - if you are splurging a little and not worried about the budget
5. Avocado
6. Cut up onions

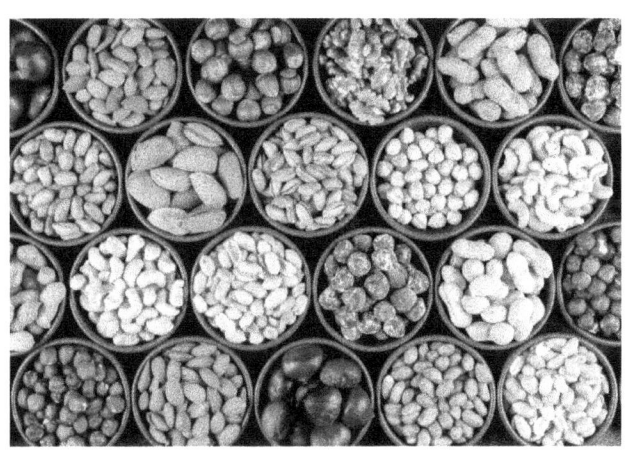

SEEDS

For the Lord your God is bringing you into a good land, a land of brooks of water, of fountains and springs, flowing out in the valleys and hills, a land of wheat and barley, of vines and fig trees and pomegranates, a land of olive trees and honey. Deuteronomy 8:7-8

Day 8:

Scripture Reading: Genesis 1:28-32, Matthew 13:3-8

Behold, I have given you every plant yielding seed that is on the face of all the earth, and every tree with seed in its fruit. You shall have them for food.
Genesis 1:29

Seeds. God gave us teeny tiny little things called seeds; seeds to sow, seeds to plant, seeds to spread throughout the earth. He could have given us anything: tractors, the internet, shopping malls. But, on day six of the creation of the world, he chose to give us seeds. Our seeds need to be in fertile soil in order to grow. How fertile is your soil? Are there things that you need to do to tend to your soil? Remove the weeds. Add nutrients? Let's spend today imagining your body and spirit as soil.

Let's do an exercise and spend a little time reflecting on our soil. In every untended soil, there are weeds. In our reading passages today in Matthew 13:7, Jesus was referring to weeds; our seeds falling among the weeds and being choked out. Our weeds reflect sin. Below, just briefly jot out few sins that you struggle with frequently. If you want to keep these private, just write the first letter of the word. God knows what is on your heart.

_____

_____

_____

Nichole Fogleman

Sometimes weeds extend from other soil. Your neighbor's weeds may have passed over into your garden and spoiled your patch of earth. Maybe some weeds have passed from generation to generation. One weed was passed to my soil from the gardens of the home on the lake with the fruit trees. From now on we will refer to this place as (H-LFT). This place is central to my understanding as a human being and we will come back here often throughout the pages of this book.

The weeds from H-LFT were passed down from generation to generation. They were embedded into my soil. They wrapped themselves around three generations of believers and tried to pull me literally under the water. I was drowning figuratively when God spoke to me under the water while I was floating in a pool. My sin was drowning me. He reached in and plucked the weed right out of my soil. As He pulled, I surrendered, and He supported my garden as I continued to cultivate the soil. He saved me from the destruction of life and family. Eventually, I renounced the generational choking weed from being passed down to the generations that I was nurturing, my two daughters. Generational sin can be stopped, whether it's alcohol, adultery, unforgiveness, or greed. The Creator of this earth can flush out soil and start anew. He has the power. Sometimes one only needs to recognize and ask.

I continue to cultivate this patch of soil in my garden today. It's taken almost 15 years to nourish and fertilize this plot of land, but I feel God planting new seeds now. *After sharing my story, again I ask, are there weeds you need to pull? Go back to the exercise above and scribble some thoughts.*

Today's Tip: Foods that Heal.
For years I have worked or been associated with our local academic hospital. Interestingly, scientists have facilitated the study of Vitamin

C for treating a wide range of medical diagnoses, from sepsis, and traumatic brain injury, to multi-organ failure. (1) Vitamin C is proven in animal models to heal. Many studies have been conducted worldwide with a wide variety of successes in the human model.

What they do know is that Vitamin C is an antioxidant, has anti-inflammatory properties, and works to eliminate free radicals. In a study evaluating Vit C for use in musculoskeletal injuries, Barker et al., (2) recommend that a "baseline vitamin C status was associated with beneficial outcomes in strength, suggesting that long-term dietary habits are more effective than short-term supplements." What are the recommended doses of Vitamin C? The recommended dietary allowance for healthy individuals is 75mg and 90mg per day for women and men. (3) However, scientists are now recommending 200 mg per day to reap the benefits of the healing properties of Vitamin C. (4)

So, if we settle with the theory of Barker et al. (2) that "long-term dietary habits are more effective than short-term supplements" let's extrapolate that into including fruits and vegetables that are high in Vitamin C in our diets during our 40-day journey. (5,6)

 Kiwi - 75 mg
 Strawberries - 95 mg
 Cantaloupe - 60 mg
 Broccoli - 60 mg
 Kale - 55 mg
 Peppers - 65 mg
 Fermented cabbage (sauerkraut) - higher than most fresh Vegetables
 Potatoes - 25 mg
 Cabbage - 20 mg
 Cauliflower - 25 mg
 Snow peas - 40 mg

Day 9:

Scripture Reading: Deuteronomy 8:1-10

The whole commandment that I command you today you shall be careful to do, that you may live and multiply, and go in and possess the land that the Lord swore to give to your fathers. Deuteronomy 8:1

The seeds that our creator gave us on the sixth day are ready to be used, the seed of wild grass, cultivated into wheat. The Israelites had spent forty years in the wilderness completely relying on God. He provided manna to eat. But it was time for them to take the next step in their journey to the promised land; "*a land of brooks of water, of fountains and springs, flowing out in the valleys and hills, a land of wheat and barley, of vines and fig trees and pomegranates, a land of olive trees and honey, a land in which you will eat bread without scarcity, in which you will lack nothing, a land whose stones are iron, and out of whose hills you can dig copper.*" (Deuteronomy 8:8) To make bread with wheat required productivity. God was ready to work through them, not just have them rely on Him.

Are you still living in the wilderness? If you are, God has made promises that we can rely on. I think back about my mom and her relentless pain. She once had a young man living with her; he was in the middle of a divorce and had nowhere to go. My mom took him in. After some time, she had to ask him to leave. She was so embarrassed by her screams in the middle of the night from her disparaging pain.

After my mother passed on, I sorted through all the books she had read. She was one of those people that took notes and wrote all along the margins. I learned more about her life in those margins than I had learned in a lifetime. One of the comments she made in a book about the hardships of pain by V.G. Beers, was "My life" and she drew an arrow to the following paragraph. "I don't like to be broken any more than you. But when I am broken, I want God to release life-giving gifts for the healing of other broken people around me. When you are broken, ask how you can grace the life of someone else through this experience." (7) My mom was in her wilderness, trying to live these words.

Spend some time today surveying your life. I ask again, are you currently living in the wilderness? Do you have a loved one living in the wilderness? While in the wilderness, He will take care of you and give you manna when the need is there, but at some point, He will be ready for you to move on, and use those seeds He provided to make bread. On the lines below, jot down briefly those people in your life that are broken; your neighbor, your sister, your husband. Let's live out actively the words above, "when you are broken, ask how you can grace the life of someone else through your experiences." (7)

Do one thing special for that person today; write them a note, give them a call, or just tell them that you love them.

_____

_____

_____

_____

Today's Tip: Foods That Heal

It's easy to make recommendations by extrapolating data from scientific studies. But what about using the diet for healing for real people? I have done a few studies on myself over the years, from healing my gut after a horrible incident with Aleve, to healing after a double mastectomy with breast cancer, and healing after reconstructive Achilles tendon surgery. There is no microscope to peer into the depths of my cells, but anecdotally I can describe healing from all of these with outstanding results. Most recently, I'm now running 8 miles a week with sprints and hill work one year after the Achilles reconstruction, never thinking I would run again. What were some of the things I did to heal?

Neal Barnard, author of Food for Life wrote a fabulous book called "Foods That Fight Pain" (8). After the most recent surgery, I scoured his book and incorporated the following into my daily regimen for three months.

Increased the amount of ALA (alpha-linolenic acid) in my diet. These fight inflammation and can be found in beans (navy, pinto, lima), citrus fruit, wheat germ, and especially in flaxseed oil. (8) I used 1 tsp. of cold flaxseed oil per day in foods and/or take a flaxseed oil supplement and added 1 tsp ground flaxseed to oatmeal. Flaxseed is also rich in Omega- 3.

I also increased the amount of GLA (gamma-linolenic acid) in my diet. These also fight inflammation (8). I took a supplement of Evening Primrose Oil 300 mg daily and added 1 tsp of Hemp to the oatmeal breakfast bowl daily.

I began taking a Vitamin B 6 supplement - 150 mg per day. This supplement has shown promise and may have benefits for chronic headaches, depression, premenstrual syndrome (PMS), carpal tunnel syndrome, and back pain. (8) Avoid doses higher than 200mg - could be associated with nerve damage. ** (8)

Lastly, I increased the number of foods high in magnesium. See Day 11, for more about the benefits of magnesium.

Along with a physical regimen prescribed by the surgeon and physical therapists, things progressed well. It was slow going, but with patience, the results were worth the wait.

** Any time you begin a diet or take a supplementation regimen, it is recommended to consult your medical doctor**

Day 10:

Scripture Reading: John 12:20-26, Ruth 3:1-18

Truly, truly, I say to you, unless a grain of wheat falls into the earth and dies, it remains alone; but if it dies, it bears much fruit. John 12:24

Ready to make bread? Still spending time in the margins of books, this time it's my mother's words written in the margins, "I have to be broken to free my life-giving gifts to those around me," In our scripture reading, Jesus was teaching his disciples that in order to bear fruit they must also die to this world and revealing mysteries about his preeminent death. My mom was learning this lesson. Her life, as she began to depend on God, became noticeably different. I could see her soul change. I could see her spirit change. Only now after she has passed, do I get to see the full evidence of her transformation as I sift through her belongings.

The seeds planted, the soil cultivated, the harvest fulfilled. The soil must be broken to free its nutrients. We go to the garden, put our hands in the soil and break up the clumps of dirt to improve the bounty of our harvest. "The wheat plants yield their grain best when they are cut and mutilated, the wheat grain yields flour most when crushed," lessons learned from the author of mom's book by V. Gilbert Beers (7)

There's an ancient story about a place where wheat plants were crushed and mutilated. A redemption story. The place where wheat was trampled often by cattle or oxen on a threshing floor. This trampling helped loosen the grain so it could be harvested. On a special night in history, Ruth, the ancestor of Jesus took a risk and met her redeemer, Boaz, on the threshing floor. The words Ruth whispered to Boaz that night on the threshing floor, ring true to us today. (10,11) "I am your servant _____, for you are my family redeemer." (Ruth 3:8) Fill in the blank with your name. The family redeemer today is Jesus, our Lord and savior.

There is another book I found long ago... In this book, I was the one that took notes and wrote in the margins. This book was my grandmother's book. The title of the book, *"The Girl's Still Got it. Take a Walk with Ruth and the God who Rocked her World."* (10) I was so intrigued that my grandmother had read this book, the same author that wrote, *"Bad Girls of the Bible"* "Meme," what were you reading? After she died, I sifted through her book and surprisingly found Ruth's story of redemption. Through the testimony of this book, I realized then that my family could be redeemed. In the margins of my grandmother's book, I underlined this quote, "When we are down to almost nothing, God is up to something bigger than we can ever imagine." (10) He is our family redeemer. We, these forty days, are preparing ourselves for something bigger than we can ever imagine. I needed this lesson today; I hope you did too.

I end today with one more word about the threshing of wheat. There are mysteries in these words spoken long ago by John the Baptist. He was speaking about Jesus and those that would be future believers in Christ. *"His winnowing fork is in his hand, and he will clear his threshing floor, gathering his wheat into the barn and burning up the chaff with unquenchable fire." (Matthew 3:12)* When he clears his threshing floor, we want to make sure we are the wheat that falls back to the ground to be harvested and not the chaff.

Today's Tip: Vitamin B - 12
A diet including only plants requires taking one very important supplement, Vitamin B-12. Vitamin B-12 is derived mostly from animals. The main sources of vitamin B-12 for humans in a

nonvegetarian diet of meat, fish, milk, cheese, and eggs; all the foods we are avoiding. (12,13)

Dr. Bernard of *Foods That Fight Pain* recommends taking 5 mcg or more per day. (8)

The supplement is usually refrigerated. I use the dropper form that goes under the tongue and take 5,000 mcg weekly in one dose. One study did find that taking a daily sublingual dose of 5 mcg is better than doing a weekly dose. (14) Maybe I'll adjust my dosing after this research.

Why does it matter? What harm can occur if I do not take this vitamin? A diet lacking in Vitamin 12 can be associated with nervous system problems; peripheral neuropathy, and memory loss.

Day 11:

Scripture Reading: Genesis 17:5-8, Acts 3:24-25, Galatians 3:29

You are the sons of the prophets and of the covenant that God made with your fathers, saying to Abraham, 'And in your seed shall all the families of the earth be blessed.' Acts 3:25

Seeds were sown at the house by the lake, (H-LFT). Seeds, which contained the kernel of my soul, were spread to myself and ultimately to future generations. Spending season after season at H-LFT, I learned about God, not entirely from the people that lived there, but from the house of worship just down the street. The people in that house knew God, and their relationship with Him prospered through trials and tribulations later in life, but while I lived in this little town, most of the gifts I received were from seeds.

On an unofficial day in 1978, in a little church down the street from H-LFT, during a hell fire damnation sermon at a revival in the south during the great evangelical revolution (See the movie "Woodlawn." This was my life.) I heard the audible voice of God and I ran. Remembering like it was yesterday, this moment forever changed my story. The seeds that were planted began to sprout.

The word used for seed in Genesis 1:28-32, the verses introduced on day 1 of this week, was the Hebrew word *zara*. (15) The word for seed translated into Greek in Galatians and Acts was *sperma*. Our text originates from the Old Testament and the New Testament, the Old Testament written in Hebrew, and the New Testament written in Greek. The word, *zara* or *sperma*, refers to seeds like we use to grow grain, or it can refer to the word for offspring, and descendants. As we

In the Garden

tie it all together, on Day 6 God gave man seed; seed to eat, and seed to produce offspring.

The promise given to Abraham in Genesis 17:5-8 was a promise about seeds *(Zara- Hebrew) These* seeds represent offspring that were guaranteed the promises from our heavenly father. In Galatians 3:29 it states, "if you belong to Christ, then you are Abrams's *seed (sperma-Greek)*, heirs according to the promise." I became an heir to Abraham's seed (zara- Hebrew) on that day in 1978. The same seed *(zara-Hebrew)* God created on Day 6. Instead of sowing seeds into the soil, He was sowing seeds into my heart.

If you have made it this far in our journey, God has already been planting seeds for you to spread. Take a few moments today and ask God to reveal those seeds to you. Are they about spreading seeds to future generations or more intimately are they about the seeds He has planted in you?

Today's Tip: Foods High in Magnesium

On day 8 I briefly spoke about adding foods high in magnesium to your diet and wanted to expound further on this topic. Since the peak of the opioid epidemic, the profession of anesthesia, the profession I work in daily, has developed protocols incorporating substitutes for medications that are helpful with pain, trying to limit the use of opioids. We call this a multi-modal approach. Magnesium is one of the medications we use. Without getting into the complicated scientific details, magnesium helps with the actions of regulating one of the receptors that regulate pain. (16)

Which foods can we introduce into our diet that are high in magnesium? (17)

    Barley - 158 mg (consistency similar to rice or quinoa)
    Brown rice - 86 mg
    Chickpeas - 78 mg
    Dried Figs - 111 mg (Amos would love this tip!)
    Northern Beans - 88 mg
    Lentils - 71 mg
    Lima Beans - 82 mg
    Navy Beans -107 mg
    Oatmeal - 70 mg
    Soybeans - 148 mg
    Spinach - 158 mg
    Tofu - 118 mg
    Swiss Chard - 152 mg

Taking a supplement is not recommended if eating quantities of the recommended foods above, especially if you are eating beans and drinking organic soy daily. Magnesium has also been shown to be beneficial to the treatment of migraines. (18) If you are counting milligrams in your food intake shoot for 400 - 700 mg per day.

Day 12:

Scripture Reading: Luke 17: 1-6, Mark 4:30-32

If you had faith like a grain of mustard seed, you could say to this sycamore tree 'Be uprooted and planted in the sea.' and it would obey you. Luke 17: 5-6

God is the master gardener. It blows me away to think about every detail of every tree, every plant, every seed, He spoke into being. Christ knew when he was standing there talking with the disciples as they were asking him to "increase their faith," that the tree (possibly the same species as the beloved sycamore-fig tree) amongst Him hailed a very aggressive root system keeping it anchored into the ground. And then in Mark 4:30-32, Jesus spoke with in-depth knowledge about the mustard seed and its size and growth pattern. All of life started in a garden.

As you read today's scripture, circle the text that speaks to you. Every scripture, and every word will speak to you differently, at a different time. This is how you practice hearing God's voice. One of God's promises was to grant us a helper to understand His word. "He will teach you all things" (John 14:26) The lines below are for you to rewrite the words, the sentences that stand out to you at this moment from Luke 17:1-6. Meditating on God's word should be about "pondering, personalizing, and practicing Scripture," according to biblical meditation expert, Robert J. Morgan. (19)

_____

_____

Nichole Fogleman

The words I write in this book are to help you the reader on your journey with chronic illness. I share advice from my life, tips from experts, and a method to bring it all together. Reading the Bible regularly is life-changing. I see how it works in my own life, and I do not suffer from a debilitating disease. I can only imagine what life would look like without God's assistance. Reading, studying, and meditating on God's word should be a practice you take with you for the rest of your life, not just these 40 days. Paul says, "Let God's word dwell in you." Read the wise words of Charles Spurgeon from one of his sermons written in the 1800s., (20)

> *"In order that it may dwell in you, it must first enter into you. You must really know the spiritual meaning of it; you must believe it; you must live upon it; you must drink it in; you must let it soak into your innermost being. It is not enough to have a bible on the shelf; it is infinitely better to have its truths stored up within your soul"*

Honestly, I struggle with memorizing scripture. I have always been so impressed by those that can study, memorize, and quote full passages. It hasn't been for the lack of trying, carrying around Bible memory verses with me in my wallet or in the car; it doesn't come naturally. Meditation is not a thing that flows naturally for me either. Things that I have done to help: taking a warm bath while meditating in complete isolation, listening to meditative music from Spa radio or

In the Garden

"Inspired Chill" music from Apple Music, or an app called Abide Bible Prayer Meditation. There are more and more tools out there now. Psychologists have figured out what ancient prophets knew thousands of years ago, meditating on God's word is paramount for mental health.

Today's Tip: Pineapples

I learned the following tips from a favorite book and from the athlete, Scott Jurek. Pineapple has a pain-fighting anti-inflammatory chemical called bromelain. Bromelain was discovered centuries ago and has been used by many populations to treat pain and for its impact to fight inflammation. The chemical structure is similar to substances used to make aspirin and ibuprofen. Most bromelain is contained in the stem of the pineapple. (21,22) Here's what I do; cut the pineapple. Eat the fruit of the pineapple for the vitamin C levels (25 mg) and cut the stem into small pieces. Place in a bag and snack on these throughout the day.

Day 13:

Scripture Reading: Psalms 126

Those who go out weeping,
carrying seed to sow,
will return with songs of joy,
carrying sheaves with them. Psalm 126:6

Worship without music is like a void of nothingness to my soul. Psalm 126 may have been a song the Israelites sang during the harvest of their fruits, the harvest of the productive seed. Hearing God's word spoken through song can be just as powerful as reading it. Today we are going to spend some time meditating in worship with music. You pick the music; old CDs or a track on Spotify.

One of my favorite songs is written in the first person as if God was speaking directly to me. During a very difficult season, I would listen to this song over and over again to feed my soul, imaging God wrapping his arms around me. Recently I found a new song using the same technique. The song is called "Love Song" by UpperRoom. It's so beautiful. Undoubtedly the worship band wrote the song amid our world shutdown, during COVID, during a 40-day fast. Wow, what 40 days can do.

The lyrics that spoke to me apply directly to our study. It's so cool how life works when you are listening to God's voice.

"I'm bringing you back to the garden. Back where it all started. All of your sins have been pardoned. Now we just get to be together."

In the Garden

On our last day together this week, let's end with an image of these beautiful lyrics. During these 40 days, your savior is bringing you back to the garden, before, the 1st man and woman had to take the leaves from the fig trees and place them over their naked bodies. He's bringing you back where it all started, where our souls were healed, and our spirits were one with his. And for the next 27 days, we just "get to be together."

Place the song you picked on repeat, go to that place in your mind that brings up the peace and spend quality time today with your savior, visualizing the words in the song or the words from our scripture reading. If you do have a Spotify account, Hope for Pain has created a Christian Meditation playlist for this bible study at *https://open.spotify.com/playlist/6eax9QE1q6uN1kXvyeawI1*.

Create a Spotify account for free and type in the link. Enjoy.

Today's Tip: Turmeric

Another important anti-inflammatory chemical found in food is curcumin, a substance in turmeric, which works to help diminish symptoms of joint pains. "By sprinkling black pepper on your curry, you increase the bioavailability of curcumin by 2,000 percent, states Dr. Will Bulsiewicz, author of New York Times Best Seller, *Fiber Fueled, The Plant-Based Gut Health Program. (23)*" Curcumin is an antioxidant, anti-cancer, and antimicrobial. At the cellular level, it blocks the activation of NF-B activation, a pathway, that signals inflammation. (24,25)

My favorite method of consuming Turmeric is by Soymilk Turmeric Latte, also called "Golden Milk." Take 1 cup of organic soymilk, and warm on stove top gently over low heat, stirring often. As the milk begins to warm add 1/2 tsp of Turmeric and a pinch of black pepper and stir. I own a small hand frother, called Aerolatte Milk Frother purchased on amazon for $21. Make your latte for pennies a year.

Day 14:

Day of Rest

In the Garden

The Simple Baked Potato

Potatoes have unfairly gotten a bad rap. They are very good for you, full of nutrients, and important microbes for your gut. Potatoes have 11% protein and 0% fat are high in fiber and contain high levels of Vitamin C. "Potatoes contain resistant starch and resistant starch is wonderful for the gut microbiome." according to health expert Dr. Will Bulsiewicz (23) author of Fiber Fueled, an amazing resource to collect as you eat more plants. Dr, B. as his friends call him, has developed an app counting plants. The more you eat the healthier your gut.

Ingredients:

Russet potato
Lemon
Sea salt

Procedure:

Wrap the potato in parchment paper and poke several holes in the potato after it's wrapped. Bake at 350 degrees for 1 to 1 1/2 hours. The test to see if your potato is ready includes squeezing the potato to make sure it's nice and soft. Unwrap your potato once it's done. Squeeze the juice of the lemon over the potato and add a little salt. No butter is needed. No sour cream is needed. Just deliciousness.

THE FORMER AND LATTER RAIN

I will give you rain for your land in tis season, the early rain and the latter rain, that you may gather in your grain, your new win and your oil. Deuteronomy 11:14

Day 15:

Scripture Reading: Deuteronomy 8:1-18

Be careful to follow every command I am giving you today, so that you may live and increase and may enter and possess the land the Lord promised...
Deuteronomy 8:1

Moses instructed the Israelites to "carefully follow the terms of a covenant, so that they may prosper in everything they did." Covenant, the word used in these verses indicated a ritual concerning obedience, which theologically indicates an agreement made involving a relationship between God and his people, with the relationship being the key word. In Deuteronomy 8:9, Moses told the Israelites that their Lord was bringing them into a good land, a land in which they would eat bread without scarcity, in which they would lack nothing. This promise is also meant for you, and this new land includes relationships, a relationship with the God almighty.

This week we will spend time talking about how to water our fertile soil in the promised land. But before we water our soil let's spend some time thinking about promises. Have there been promises that others have made to you and then let you down? Have you made promises to friends or family that you have not fulfilled? The lines below are to help guide you to make a list of unfilled hopes and dreams relating to your relationship with God. I have given you an illustration to get you started. Have fun with this.

Unfulfilled Hopes	Hope for the Future
1. I heard your voice incorrectly and made a mess of things.	1. I hear your voice correctly

While on this earth God intended for us to have a relationship with him, this is part of his promises. God's promises are not exclusively about getting to heaven, it's about living the life we are supposed to live while on earth, and then when our lives are done here, we get to spend eternity with Him. God places hopes and dreams in our hearts for us to thrive here on this planet. Just as our parents want us to thrive out in the world after we graduate from high school, of course not all of us are blessed with great parents, and I'm not naive to think that this is common ground, but theoretically good parents want everything for their children: purposeful life, benevolent relationships, and they want to talk on the phone with them at least every other day to hear how things are going. Our Heavenly Father is no different. You are graduating from high school and it's time to dream. And keep in touch with dad to let him know how things are going and what you need to keep adversity and challenges at bay.

But don't forget when you leave high school and get that fabulous job you always dreamed of and sit in the theoretical beach chair next to your gorgeous house on the beach, not to neglect Moses warning in verse 17, "When you have eaten your fill, be sure to praise the Lord your God for the good land he has given you."

Today's Tip: Food Journal
We are in week three of this journey. You most likely are seeing some changes, feeling some changes. It can be a lot to take in and absorb. This week we are going to start a food journal. At the back of the book is a resource I created for you. If you are one of those people that read the back of the book and found the food journal chart and already started this, then kudos to you!! Journaling your food progression can be immensely helpful in pinpointing which foods are tolerated or not. Make a copy or record it in the notes section of your phone. Include the following: The time of day you eat. Your mood when you eat. Your sensation of hunger. The actual food. We are going to start counting plant points. Plant points are a concept created by Dr. B. in the book *Fiber Fueled. (1)* There is even an app that was created called Nibble to count plant points. The more points per day the better. For us it's more about the journey, challenging you to look more at what you are eating and how you feel. To record points, I want you to only record 1 point per food item. If you eat oatmeal with blueberries, flaxseed, hemp, walnuts, and soymilk then that counts as 6 points. The last thing you will be recording is your symptoms. Do you feel bloated every time you eat a piece of whole grain toast?

Nichole Fogleman

What will we do with these journals? There are no grades at the end. This is a healing journey. *"Knowledge is like a garden; if it is not cultivated, it cannot be harvested."* African Proverb

Day 16:

Scripture Reading: Deuteronomy 11:1-17

I will give you rain for your land in its season, the early rain and the latter rain, that you may gather in your grain, your new wine and your oil.
Deuteronomy 11:14

The new terrain of the Israelites was arid, unlike what they were used to in Egypt. They would have to learn new farming practices, no longer able to rely on their ancestor's knowledge, since they had been in the wilderness for 40 years. God was teaching them about their new land, a territory where they would have to be productive, *"a land that the Lord your God cares for. The eyes of the Lord your God are always upon it, from the beginning of the year to the end of the year."* (Deuteronomy11: 12) A terrain that was dependent on the former and latter rains in order to grow crops.

Wendell Berry, in *Scripture, Culture, and Agriculture,* (2) warns Americans about acquiring entitlement feelings comparing ourselves to the Israelites and our destiny to the promised land. The Israelites were left with explicit instructions to take care of the land, ecologically and agriculturally. When Israelites lived in Egypt, the land was easy to work with and when they moved to the hill country of Judah and Samaria, the land was a vast new development. Author, Wendell Berry when describing Davis's book to the reader stated "what would America be now if we white people had managed to bring with us, not just a Holy land spirituality, but also the elaborate land ethic, land reverence, and agrarian practice meant to safeguard the holiness of the land." Are we not supposed to hold the same reverence for our bodies, our lives, and our purpose today? If these things metaphorically symbolize the promised land, then I believe we are called to hold the

Nichole Fogleman

same practice. We cultivate our soil which is our soul with His Word, we plant with reverence food into our bodies and we patiently wait for God to water our seeds, resulting in nourished and healthy physical bodies.

There will be seasons that require patience, times when it feels like the rains are never going to come. But He promises to bring the rain. There is a warning in our new land in verses 16. *"Be careful, or you will be enticed to turn away and worship other gods and bow down to them. Then the Lord's anger will burn against you, and he will shut up the heavens so that it will not rain and the ground will yield no produce, and you will soon perish from the good land the Lord is giving you."* (The Message) We do not want to go through a season of famine ever again. We are done with the old. We are ready to move forward to our promised land, where the rain comes in a timely fashion, just when our souls and our physical bodies need refreshing.

Let's end the day with an exercise to refresh our minds with the covenant given to God's children in their new land. Write verses 13 and 14 in your own words, as if it was a prayer, making it personal between just you and God. Make it your own; sing it, write it out in your calendar, or hang it on the bathroom mirror.

_____

_____

_____

_____

_____

_____

_____

In the Garden

Today's Tip: Family Dinner
We have been eating plant-based for several years. Our children are not so gung-ho about the program, with the understanding to adjust our menus to include variety. Most of the time I try to create dinners that feature creations from both spectrums. Doesn't everyone have pizza night? We always make our pizzas. I purchase premade whole grain crusts, create pizzas the kids like, and then make a no cheese or cashew cheese for our pizza. Actually, after eating pizza with just tomato sauce and veggies cooked on the grill, I have started getting away from the extra calories and fat brought about by the cashew cheeses.

Other ideas for family meals: taco night with tortillas and beans for you and your family's favorite meat for them with lots of added-on veggies or homemade black beans burgers for everyone. Let the kids help make the burgers. We taught ourselves to make veggie sushi a few years ago. We have had a few family nights making sushi together. Get creative.

Day 17:

Scripture Reading: Matthew 7: 24-28

And the rain fell, and the floods came, and the winds blew and beat on that house, but it did not fall, because it had been founded on the rock. Matthew 7:25

When those rains come, make sure your foundation is solid. The rains will descend, and they may feel like torrential downpours. The rain He promised, the rain of former and latter days, to water our soul may come even in the form of a flood. Jesus warns us that we have to be ready, our foundations have to be solid. They have to be like a stone. To make our foundations solid, we have to be doers of the word, not just hearers; *"whoever hears my words and does them is like a wise man who builds his house on the rock."* (verse 26) The wise man's house does not fall even when the floods come.

I guarantee you that storms will come. They may feel like floods; the upstairs bathroom water starts seeping through the ceiling, the power goes off right when you are packed and leaving for a trip across the world, and the cat throws up on the leather couch right before the whole family arrives to stay for a week. You feel in the blank. What was your last flood like?

_____

_____

_____

_____

In the Garden

A hurricane of sorts impacted my world once. I was attempting to build a life on solid rock; I thought I was doing all the right things, and then boom out of nowhere that generational sin showed its way into my life from nowhere. The testing I went through, the violent storms, began as dreams. They weren't nightmares. They were lovely dreams that occurred over and over again, causing me to question my reality. At the end of my storm, I read that sometimes testing can come through dreams. Beth Moore writes in the life-changing book *When Godly People do Ungodly Things, (3)* "I did not plan on veering from the path. Nothing could have been further from my mind. I loved God with every one of my handicapped heart." At the time of my attack, I had no arsenal to protect myself. I went to church two to three times a week, taught the youth, and did all the things a good young Christian mother of two should do, and I was blindsided.

The key weapon that was missing from my life; I did not have His Word buried in my heart. Paul taught the Hebrews, "The Word of God is living, powerful, and sharper than any two-edged sword." (Hebrews 4:12) I had no sword to use in this battle. The foundation I had built my house was on sand. God's Word was the missing ingredient. I began building my foundation, and it took several years to build. It did not happen overnight. But I weathered the storm, immersed myself in His Word day and night, and haven't stopped since. It's been 15 years since the great flood of my life. Don't wait until it's too late, and the sandbags haven't been laid, and the wind begins to blow. You are taking the first step by spending these 40 days in His Word; start digging and bury it.

Today's Tip: Famer's Markets
Get out and discover your local farmer's market to find locally sourced fruits and vegetables. Oftentimes I hear the complaint that shopping at the farmer's market is cost prohibitive. Here are a few tips to make this experience more palatable. Local hospitals are beginning to run weekly farmer's markets that are affordable for patients. The institution

Nichole Fogleman

I currently work hosts a market every Wednesday and only patients are allowed to shop for the first hour. Many markets across the country now allow individuals to use their SNAP/EBT benefits (supplemental nutrition assistance program). The Farmer's Market Coalition began a program to guide markets to set up SNAP programs.[i]

    I love to shop at the market on a Saturday, only buy items for the week, and try to make only dishes with the items I buy. Great way to save money and have fun with it. Two weeks ago, we challenged ourselves to do this and had vegan pasta one night with homemade pesto, summer salads from the vegetables with corn and potatoes, black beans with homemade salsa and locally sourced tortilla chips, and vegan locally sourced burgers.

---

[i] https://farmersmarketcoalition.org/education/snap/

Day 18:

Scripture Reading: Galatians: 4:21-31, 3:28-29

And you, dear brother and sisters, are children of the promise, just like Isaac.
Galatians 4: 28

Have you ever noticed how much God's Word speaks about inheritance? It's all the over scripture, from the seed of Abraham to the chronology of Jesus, to the prodigal son. We are called to bless our seed, our biological and/or spiritual offspring with an inheritance. This inheritance is about the good news of Jesus Christ.

Let's spend a little time today unpacking inheritance and spiritual inheritance. In the gardens at H-LFT, I came to learn about inheritance. The elders that lived there, my grandparents, spoke often about this topic. It was assumed that we would all take some material items with us after they were gone. Every trip I made to their home as an adult included sending some type of item of remembrance with me so I would never forget when they leave this earth. Thank you, Meme, for the vases. I still have them.

However, the most important gift they gave to me was a heavenly inheritance. They knew the promise proclaimed in Galatians 3:2-298, *"We live in this generation, and every generation since, are his children, children born by the power of the spirit. and now that we know that we belong to Christ, we are true children of Abraham. We are his heirs, and God's promise to Abraham belongs to you."*

Now that my grandparents and their daughter, my mom, have passed, I'm so grateful for this life-changing gift they passed on to me. Today we are going to do a little exercise. I want you to write on the lines below your immediate family members: husband, wife, children, brother, sister, parents, aunt, uncle, and friends. These are your people. Do they know the Lord? They are your spiritual heirs. Or maybe you are the luckiest person in the world and everyone in your immediate family knows the Lord and they passed this inheritance to you. Take a few moments to thank these individuals and give up some gratitude today.

_____

_____

_____

_____

_____

_____

_____

_____

Today's Tip: The Plate Size Matters
This is a tip from my husband. He may have stolen it from the author of Omnivore's Dilemma, but this is one that we adopted and never looked back. We only eat on 10-inch plates. Studies have been conducted to prove or disprove the theory that the smaller the plate size the less the individual will eat, (5) One of the studies is titled "Will smaller plates lead to smaller waists?" The evidence is inconclusive, but from the Fogleman "real life" study, it works.

Day 19:

Scripture Reading: Jeremiah 3:1-5

Therefore the showers have been withheld and the spring rain has not come.
Jeremiah 3:3

During the former and the latter rain lies a period between the two when the garden is growing, producing fruit. But what if the tree stops bearing fruit, things start drying up, clouds are not forming, and there are no signs of the latter rain? In the former days, you could feel the presence of the Lord but now you feel nothing. Drought is setting in, what are you to do?

Journal briefly about a time when God's presence was lacking in your life.

_____

_____

_____

_____

_____

The words of Jeremiah from our scripture reading seem harsh but could be an indicator of the origins of our drought. These are the Words of our Lord, spoken through a man, a prophet. Have we polluted our land? Have we been polluting our bodies and our souls? Read the verses again and circle the word polluted. The word polluted in Hebrew is "chaneph," which also means "to turn to godlessness." (4)

One of the purposes of these 40 days is to rid our bodies of the toxins of this earth and begin the healing process, but also we are working to clean our souls. Years ago, our local church hosted support groups for those with chronic pain. We invited a healer to our group to perform a laying of hands ceremony. With an open mind, I observed as a lady came forward. She had chronic tinnitus, ringing in her ears. The ringing would never stop. During the ceremony, the healer stopped and asked the woman if she had sin that could be preventing her from experiencing the healing process. He stated that he could feel her sinfulness. He could feel her "chaneph," the pollution that was preventing her from being healed. She began to cry, and the latter rain began to pour. She proclaimed to feel healing at that moment as she let go of her sin. Her tears of "latter" rain cleaned out the pollution of her inner soul.

It was the first time I had witnessed anything like this but the elements of release were something I would never forget. The answer lies in the next chapter of Jeremiah 4. "The Message" translates it into beautiful, easy-to-understand terms. *"If you want to come back you must come back to me. You must get rid of your stinking sin paraphernalia and not wander away from me anymore."* We know we will wander, and most likely we will pollute our souls over and over again. But thank you God through our savior Jesus, He forgives us for this nasty pollution and gives us a route for redemption called repentance. Repenting is an act of return. In Jeremiah 3:1, the word "return" used by God means to turn back in spiritual relation to God. He desires our return.

Today's Tip: Releasing Your Aching Back With Food
Could the way you eat affect your back? The word is out that eating healthy helps fight heart disease. But what if the arteries in your spine narrowed the same as the arteries in your heart, and that was the origin

of back pain in some individuals? Studies have been conducted investigating this phenomenon (6, 7) According to Neal Bernard author of *Foods That Fight Pain (8)*, "the average person with a history of back pain was found to have two arteries to the lower back completely blocked." These were results found in autopsies. Bernard goes on to state, "could it be that back pain begins not in the back muscles or the spine but in the arteries?" To extrapolate this even further, eating a vegan diet has been proven to reverse heart disease. If there is one book I recommend for further reading, it would be Caldwell Esselstyn's book *"Prevent and Reverse Heart Disease, the Revolutionary, Scientifically Proven Nutrition-Based Cure"*. Did you catch that in the title, **Nutrition Based Cure? (9, 10)** More about this tomorrow.

Day 20:

Scripture Reading: Hosea 6: 1-3

He will come to us like the rain. Like the latter and former rain to the earth.
Hosea 6:3

The words on these pages this week have written themselves. Prior to listening to a sermon by Charles Spurgeon, (11), I had never heard of the former and latter rains. It's amazing the number of times the phrase is used in scripture. With the Israelites being an agricultural culture, the reference makes sense, but there are very few coincidences in God's Word. Words may seem literal in the Old Testament writings, and then we switch to the New Testament and the figurative language is never-ending. What have we learned this week about the former and latter rains? Rewrite the verse from Hosea below.

_____

_____

_____

_____

Is not His Word beautiful? I am in "awe" so many times. As we touched on yesterday, the Lord wants us to return, and repent. Things have felt hard, but He wants to heal. He is ready to revive us, to raise us; like He did his own son. We must live in His ways. During the in-between times, between the former and latter rains, we are to work on our foundations making them strong, reading His Word, studying His Word, "being doers, not just hearers," and most importantly burying His Word in our hearts so we always have it there for those rough in-between days. Thank you, Hosea. Thank you, God.

> *"Come, let us return to the Lord;*
> *for he has torn us, that he may heal us;*
> *he has struck us down, and he will bind us up.*
> *After two days he will revive us;*
> *on the third day, he will raise us,*
> *that we may live before him.*
> *Let us know; let us press on to know the Lord;*
> *his going out is sure as the dawn;*
> *he will come to us as the showers,*
> *as the spring rains that water the earth."*
> Hosea 6:1-3

Today's Tip: Nutrition-Based Cure
Dr. Esselstyn, the author of the *Nutrition Based Cure* mentioned on day 19, studied 17 individuals, for over five years, placed them on a plant-based diet, and reversed their heart disease. (10) In his book, he wrote that many of his patients told him how difficult it is to change and maintain this diet. He believes that after "twelve weeks of eating no animal foods, dairy, or added oils, you lose your craving for fat." (9) Your palate changes. You begin to taste the spices in foods and the natural flavors. This is not a myth. This is a fact. It's like learning to smell the nuances of wine from a sommelier. Your senses change from the tongue to the olfactory cells in your nose. You will begin to crave healthy food.

Day 21:

Your Day of Rest

Recipe

Let's make some bread. Cornbread, a southern favorite, goes well with any beans. This recipe was adapted from a gluten-free recipe using brown rice flour. I've made it for the most southern discerning palates that love the taste of fat buttery bread, and they thought it was fabulous.

Plant-Based Corn Bread

Ingredients:

1 cup brown rice flour
3/4 cup cornmeal
3 tbs sugar
2 1/2 tsp baking powder
1 tsp sea salt
2 vegan flax eggs
1 cup non-dairy milk - I use rice milk
1/4 cup melted vegan butter - I use Earth Balance

Procedure:

Preheat the oven to 400 degrees. Mix flour, cornmeal, sugar, baking powder, and salt together in a medium bowl. In a small bowl, mix flaxseed eggs, milk, and 1/4 cup of the vegan butter. To make flaxseed eggs, use 1 Tbs of ground flaxseed and mix with 3 Tbs of water. Do this twice to make two eggs. Place in the refrigerator for 15 minutes or 10 minutes in the freezer. Combine both mixtures and stir to just moisten. Pour batter into your favorite pan to bake cornbread. In the south, we often use cast iron. Bake for 15- 20 minutes. Serve warm.

THE FRUIT OF THE SPIRIT

The fruit of the Spirit is love, joy, peace, patience, kindness, goodness, faithfulness, gentleness, and self-control; against such things, there is no law. Galatians 5:22-23

Day 22:

Scripture Reading: John 15:1-8

Every branch in me that does not bear fruit he takes away, and every branch that does bear fruit he prunes, that it may bear more fruit. John 15:2

You have made it! You are halfway there. In our scripture today, we move into the garden, with a reminder that God is our gardener. No longer are we the "dresser" of fruit. In the New King James Version of the Bible, it states that God is now our vinedresser. In verse 3 of John 15, it reminds us that now that we have faith in Christ, we are clean because of God's Word.

The night before Jesus was arrested, He told his disciples the story of the vine and the branches. Only the gospel of John shares this story. John was there sitting at the table with Jesus. It's easy to overlook these verses and move on. There are so many things Jesus was sharing with them that evening. But this parable must have had utmost importance, as he sandwiched it between his explanations about the Holy Spirit. And maybe that's the point. He is pruning us to bear the fruits of the spirit. We are told in Galatians 5:22-23 that the Holy Spirit gives us the fruit of the spirit.

Today let's do a quick exercise. Glimpse over Galatians 5:22-23, *"But the fruit of the Spirit is love, joy, peace, patience, kindness, goodness, faithfulness, gentleness, self-control; against such things, there is no law"* We will spend the rest of the week unpacking this verse. Make a list below of those qualities you embrace and those that you struggle with.

No problem, I've got this! "Joy"
The struggling Fruit, I do not have this! "Love"

Me: Joy   Me: Love

You: _____   You: _____

Today's Tip: To Oil or Not to Oil
There is a confusing advice about the consumption of oil. The Mediterranean diet proclaims that olive oil consumption is just fine. Dr. Esselstyn completely restricts oil of any kind. Interestingly I have played around with learning how to cook without oil. There are many great techniques for this process. The organization "Forks over Knives" does a great job illustrating this concept.[ii]

They recommend using stainless steel pans, cast iron, or ceramic titanium. We use the *Green Pan*, nonstick cookware, easily find it on Amazon for $49 for two pans. Other recommendations include using parchment paper when roasting and no oil. On the Hope for Pain plan, I allow grapeseed oil for cooking and flax-seed oil for noncooking recipes. Grapeseed has a very high smoking point leading to fewer toxins and may have some beneficial components as an anti-inflammatory agent. If using oil, use a small amount, 1 tsp at the most, and try some of the techniques described on the website given below. I do use very small amounts of vegan butter occasionally for baking.

[ii] https://www.forksoverknives.com/wellness/plant-based-cooking-how-to-cook-without-oil.

Day 23:

LOVE

Scripture Reading: Galatians 5:22-26, Deuteronomy 10:12

What does the Lord your God require of you, but to fear the Lord your God, to walk in all his ways, to love him, to serve the Lord your God with all your heart and with all your soul. Deuteronomy 10:12

My Bible titles this section of Galatians as "Living by the Spirit Power." Paul the writer of Galatians remarks as if speaking directly to our hearts, "So I say, let the Holy Spirit guide your lives." Today we are going to let Him guide us on how to love.

We all come to this circle with different stories, and different circumstances; married, divorced, orphaned, adopted, mother, father, sister, brother. Maybe we tried to love others, but our hearts were trampled. This time when we practice loving others, we will have a guide, an advocate, in our corners. We only have to place ourselves out there, allow Him to prune our branches, and then we will start bearing more fruit.

Let's start with a simple task: loving your heavenly father more today than you did yesterday. Write below the 2nd scripture (Deuteronomy 10:12) in whichever version of the bible you have.

_____

_____

_____

_____

_____

We are required to love him. Try the following exercise. Write down any reason to love Him.

He gives us the desires of our hearts. Psalm 37:4

_____

He helps when my flesh fails. Psalm 73:25

_____

He is the strength of my heart. Psalm 73:25

_____

He hears my voice and petitions. Psalm 116:1

_____

We no longer have to offer burning offering and sacrifices Mark 12:33

_____

Things work together for good, for those that love Him. Romans 8:28

_____

In the Garden

The list could go on and on. Today we are practicing how to love, to love the Creator of this universe, the all-knowing omnipresent Lord. Tomorrow we will prune our branches a little and practice loving others.

Dear Heavenly Father, loving you has never been difficult for me. I can close my eyes and feel your arms wrapping me in your embrace. But I know that others may not be able to feel this love, with the same capacity. Please Lord, work on our hearts today. Show us how to love you more, create in our souls, in our spirits a love for you that surpasses all understanding. Amen.

Today's Tip: What About those Salty or Sweet Cravings?
The following snacks are tried and true favorites at the Fogleman household: Frozen Grapes and Air-popped popcorn.

Sweet craving: Frozen Grapes. There is a technique to the process. Take red grapes and wash them. Lay them out sorted off the vine onto paper towels and allow them to dry. Use 1-quart storage bins to create small portions and place grapes in bins and freeze for 24 hours. Enjoy any time you need a sweet snack. Warning. They are addictive.

Salty Craving: Air Popped Popcorn. This does require a small expense of purchasing an air popper ($23 on Amazon) but is truly a satisfying snack to fulfill the salty craving. Pop the organic corn with no oil in the popper then add spray Bragg liquid amino and nutritional yeast. The fun part of cooking is experimenting. Spray the Bragg liquid amino and add the nutritional yeast to your liking.

Day 24:

LOVE

Scripture Reading: Matthew 22: 34-40, 1 Corinthians 13:1-8

Love your neighbor as you love yourself. Matthew 22:39

Today we flesh out the second part of Jesus's greatest commandment "loving others." The first part comes naturally to me, loving our heavenly father; but loving others with the same capacity that He loves us can be quite challenging. It fully requires reliance on the promised Holy Spirit to demonstrate the love of Christ to others.

It wasn't till several years ago, that I fully understood why. It all goes back to H-LFT, the place encompassing my childhood memories. I was the product of an unplanned, loveless communion between two individuals on a heat-inspired summer evening. Two young people barely old enough to be called adults created a human; later a backroom wedding ensued, the grandparents vowed to the parents to help care for the child, and the couple tried to love each other; but they forgot one thing, to tell the child about this deep dark secret. She spent her whole life, till middle age, not understanding the concept of love, until boom, one day the secret came out. I'm speaking in the third person, of course, that person was me. My story, not unlike so many others' stories, is not heart-wrenching compared to others, but all the same, it's my story. I believe each one of us has a story that affects how well we bear fruit; for me, it's harder to love, for you it may be difficult to master self-control or to tap into joy, But I guarantee there is a least one fruit of the spirit that brings about a struggle.

Our 2nd scripture, 1 Corinthians 13:4-8, is the words often heard at weddings. These words can help us focus on the aspects required to love others more fully like Christ. Write down each quality of love in the blanks below.

_____ _____ _____ _____

_____ _____ _____ _____

_____ _____ _____ _____

_____ _____ _____ _____

There are fifteen. Even as I write these words in my journal, I discover more about my story and how it has influenced my coping skills adopted along the way. It's a work in progress, but most importantly I know that I have to rely fully on the Holy Spirit to even begin to grasp the fruit of loving others well.

Today's Tip: Oats on the Cold Side

This is my everyday routine for breakfast. It's easy. It's packed with many nutrients and will keep you full for hours. It's served cold and takes a little getting used to, but soon nothing else satisfies in the mornings.

In a bowl add ½ cup of dry old-fashioned oatmeal, ½ cup of muesli, 1 tablespoon ground flaxseed, 1 tablespoon hemp seed, and 1 handful of seasonal fruit. Add your choice of non-dairy milk. That's it. Let it soak a little while or eat it right away. Add a little honey if you need it sweeter.

Day 25:

JOY

Scripture Reading: Isaiah 35: 1-4, Psalm 40: 1-3

He put a new song in my heart, a song of praise to our God
Psalm 40:3a

God is the utmost amazing poet. The words of Isaiah 35 bring absolute joy to my heart. Take a moment and write your favorite lines of these verses. Today we are going to be focusing on the fruit: joy.

_____

_____

_____

_____

_____

Which verse speaks to you in this passage? Is it verse 3, "With this news, strengthen those who have tired hands, and encourage those who have weak knees?" Verse 1 cries out to me this morning, "even the wilderness and desert will be glad in those days, the wasteland will rejoice and blossom with spring crocuses." But even if the wasteland and desert are ready to sing hymns of gladness, it doesn't mean that you feel the same way. I believe some individuals experience difficulty feeling joy. There are times when we all pretend like we have joy in our hearts. Maye when you hear James 1:2 "when trouble of any kind comes your way, consider it an opportunity of great joy," you cringe.

While researching joy, I discovered instances where God made his people joyful. You heard it right; He MADE them have joy. In both circumstances, the Israelites were called to celebrate the dedication of a symbol of God's provision. (Ezra 6:22 and Nehemiah 12:43). The Hebrew word is "simmeham," which means to make joyful, found in several of the Bible translations. God needed to change their hearts to feel joy. They had been in exile for 70 years in Babylon. Probably a few of them did not feel like there was a reason to celebrate. They were perhaps exhausted, skeptical, or afraid. Today ask the Holy Spirit for "simmeham," to help your soul feel joy. In the 2nd part of Ezra 22, after their "simmeham" encounter with God, it states "the joy of the people of Jerusalem could be heard far away." God, I pray that our hearts will be so full of joy that our neighbors hear us laughing.

I also included Psalm 40 in our reading today. Do you recognize these verses? Can you hear Bono belting out the melody? God can put a song in our hearts, a song of praise and joy.

If this is the fruit that you struggle with, I want you to write on a notecard the word "simmeham." This is your word. This is going to be a living word God places in your heart.

Today's tip: Good Ole Basic Water

The controversy about drinking tap water runs the gamut from low-income families afraid to drink tap water, to reports of microplastics and contaminants in the water in the United States. (1,2,3)

In our family, we do not drink tap water. We own a distiller and make distilled water daily or we use the filtered water from the refrigerator. These forty days we are ridding our body of toxins. Are the risks worth the benefits? No fluoride is added to our water. You have to weigh the risks for yourself. Our dental records are clean and studies have been shown to report good oral health for people on plant-based diets. (4)

Day 26:

PEACE

Scripture Reading: Revelations 4:1-6

....before the throne, there was as it were a sea of glass, like crystal
Revelations 4:6

Recently on a Sunday during worship, our pastor pointed out a beautiful God moment in the New Testament. He was flooded with tears as he read verse 6 of Revelations. He remarked on the symbolism brought forth in his mind when the author of Revelations wrote about "the sea of glass." These images, written by John, the friend, and disciple of Jesus, are a direct glimpse of heaven. He saw God's throne and in front was a shiny sea of glass; no waves, no turbulence, no current; just complete peace.

Sometimes we need images to focus on when searching for peace. The Holy Spirit is the source of this gift, and God created our minds where images flood our memories searching for particular peaceful situations.

As a specialist in pain, I spent a little time studying the art of hypnotism. Those that have an extreme fear of surgery or anesthesia sometimes seek help from a hypnotist to help them overcome their fears. Imagery is one of the many tools in the toolbox that a hypnotist will use. You, the patient, are led to imagine a place in your mind that brings forth complete peace and comfort. With deep breathing-led exercises, the patient is led to go to that place in their minds during fearful moments. My place during the exercise was the house on the lake among the fruit trees (H-LFT). Within the depths of my memories, I could squander up images of floating on the lake and I felt complete peace. That was the very moment I realized how much that place impacted my life. What is your place on the lake? What is your sea of glass?

On the first day of the forty days, I asked you to practice finding this place. Today I want you to go there again. Lay down, take 3 to 4 deep cleansing breath, in through your nose and out through your mouth, and find the sea of glass in your mind. It could very well be the image John has given us of heaven standing before the throne of God or it could be you and your family walking along the road at Disney World. It's your image.

Paul taught us in Philippians 4:9, *"What you have learned and received and heard and seen in me - practice these things and the God of peace will be with you."* So go and practice, find your images of peace.

Today's Tip: Smoothies
Smoothies may be one of the best ways to increase the number of plants in your diet, especially if you dislike greens. The key, in my opinion, to make any juice or smoothie delicious is to add a green apple. The flavor of the green apple contrasts with greens like kale and spinach making the perfect combination.

And if there is any financial investment you can make to this lifestyle, it is purchasing a Vitamix. The Vitamix is a game changer, an industrial type of mixer for the domestic home kitchen. It makes the creation of smoothies fun and easy. The key in my opinion is mixing the liquid and the greens first and then adding the fruits and larger vegetables. The consistency will be improved.

When we bought our Vitamix years ago, this adorable lady gave us her home recipes to try and wrote on a piece of paper the following phrase, "Vita-Mix" is a "MUST" for every home and will be a blessing in your life IF YOU USE IT. God Bless and Happy Vita-mixing. smiley Face - P.J. Who could argue with this?

In the Garden

PJ's Green Extreme

1 slice of pineapple
1 whole pear
1/2 banana
1 slice of ginger root (size of a potato chip)
1 slice lemon
1 large handful of spinach
3 tbsp honey
1 cup of vanilla soy milk
Run until smooth.

Thank you, P.J.

Day 27:

SELF CONTROL

Scripture Reading: 1 Samuel 24: 1-22, Matthew 27: 12-14, Matthew 26: 62-63

Jesus remained Silent. Matthew 26:63

There are fifteen fruits. Before we move on to the literal fruits of the vine next week, let's spend one more day in the figurative fruit of the spirit. This morning the choice was made clear after asking my spouse which fruit he has the most struggles with. His is self-control.

It's funny when searching the topical encyclopedia I use for writing, it was written in the 1800s (5), and is literally falling apart, there are only four examples of verses that speak of self-control: two are from David and two from Jesus, which seems quite fitting; David under temptation from accosting his enemy and Jesus' restraint in front of his accusers.

First, let's look at David's example. Sometimes God places tests in front of us to practice using the Holy Spirit as our advocate. Twice David was tested, being so close he could touch the cloak of his enemy, and he chose self-control. David did not always choose self-control when tested later in life when he chose to commit adultery and murder a confidant. He suffered from self-control issues. Can you think of a time when you may have been tested by God? Did you practice proper restraint or did you miserably fail? That's ok if you miserably failed because Jesus gave us the perfect example of what to do to help us practice self-control

In the Garden

This example can be found in the book of Matthew by the king almighty himself. His recipe for success when tempted to respond inappropriately; stay silent. "Jesus remained silent." This deserves a repeat. Drop the mic, Jesus.

We only covered five of the fifteen fruits. We are going to move on next week, however, if one of the other fruits speaks to you by all means do the same thing that I have done. Take that fruit, look in a bible encyclopedia or google verses with that word. Ask the Holy Spirit to speak to you and open your heart to his voice and His lessons.

Today's tips: Bananas, nuts, beans, and whole grains. What do they have in common?

These are whole foods rich in Vitamin B6, otherwise known as Pyridoxine. In 1990, several studies were conducted administering Vitamin B6 for pain. They found promising results with a reduction in lower back pain.

How does Vitamin B6 work? It works by increasing the production of neurotransmitters like dopamine, serotonin, and gamma-aminobutyric acid (GABA). Believe it or not, Vitamin B6 has been used for years to help with carpal tunnel syndrome, diabetic neuropathy, and chronic pain. Scientists found a significant reduction in back pain and lower extremity fracture pain when combined use of B6 and non-steroidal like Aleve. (6,7,8)

How much is enough? It is important to take the right dosage. Too much can be toxic. A recommended dose of B6 is 50 – 150 mg per day. Daily doses of 200 mg or higher should be avoided. Food sources rich in B6 are avocados, bananas, broccoli, brussel sprouts, chickpeas, beans, potatoes, and spinach.

When purchasing vitamins, quality is important. Visit your local natural food store to buy high-quality grade vitamins.

**Always consult your physician before beginning any new supplement.

Day 28:

Your day of Rest

In the Garden

Recipe:
Gammy's Dill Pickle Coleslaw

My Gammy was a fabulous southern cook. She made the best-fried potatoes known to man. There was one dinner in particular that she made for every special occasion which always included her coleslaw. Cabbage is a great green to keep around the house. A whole head of cabbage makes a big coleslaw to munch on throughout the week. I make a big dish for dinner one night, eat it for lunch a couple of days, and have it again for dinner.

Cabbage is extremely healthy. It is a cruciferous vegetable just like broccoli and cauliflower. Want to know the best part about cruciferous vegetables? They heal the body. Maxwell Gerson, the Moses of fighting disease with food, uses cabbage in his treatment centers. (6) Cabbage helps with memory, it is an antioxidant, and a detoxifier that has anti-inflammatory benefits and promotes healing. It's been used to treat anemia and may help with diabetes to lower blood sugar.

Ingredients:

1. Head of green cabbage - sometimes I mix red and green cabbage
2. 1 jar of dill pickles - try to find organic local pickles
3. White distilled vinegar - just buy the cheap kind
4. Sea salt
5. Pepper
6. Jar of vegan mayo (or make your own with equal parts coconut yogurt, flaxseed oil, and lemon juice) (5)
7. Red onions

Procedure:

Slice, chop, and shred the cabbage. Make it the consistency you like. A whole head of cabbage will fill a large bowl. Chop 1/2 of the red onion

Nichole Fogleman

and mix with it cabbage. Chop up three pickles into tiny pieces and mix with cabbage. In a separate container make the dressing. Mix 1 tablespoon of vegan mayo (only 1 tablespoon), if using a healthier version of homemade mayo then use more if desired. Mix mayo with 1/2 cup of pickle juice, and 1/2 cup of distilled vinegar. Add 1 tsp of sea salt to the mixture and 1/2 tsp to pepper. Then pour mixture over cabbage and blend. It's best to blend with your hands to immerse the cabbage as much as possible because you are using such a small amount of vegan mayo. Then Voila. Serve fresh or cold. I use coleslaw throughout the week and sometimes add more cabbage if needed.

THE FRUIT OF THE VINE

He dug it and cleared it of stones, and planted it with choice vines; he built a watchtower in the midst of it, and hewed out a wine vat in it; and he looked for it to yield grapes, but it yielded wild grapes.
Isaiah 5:2

Day 29:

Scripture Reading: Isaiah 5:1-2, Numbers 13: 23-24

Let me sing for my beloved
my love song concerning his vineyard:
My beloved had a vineyard
on a very fertile hill.
He dug it and cleared it of stones,
and planted it with choice vines;
he built a watchtower in the midst of it,
and hewed out a wine vat in it;
and he looked for it to yield grapes,
but it yielded wild grapes.
Isaiah 5:1-2

It's been almost 30 days. Are you starting to see and feel significant changes? We are going to spend the next six days in the vineyard. A vineyard, first seen in the promised land by Joshua and the twelve spies, who brought back a huge handful of grapes (Numbers 13: 23-24), carried on a pole to testify to the others of the fruitful bounty in the promised land.

Before moving into the promised land, the Israelites wandered for 40 years in a place called Kadesh-Barnea. Explorers in the 1800s found this barren place and documented their exploration, describing the area as completely barren of vegetation until venturing just north. According to Henry Clay Trumball, "almost immediately the long-sought wells of Qadeer were before our eyes. It was a marvelous sight!" He described venturing from a barren wasteland to a "magical suddenness" into a world of green beauty laden with fruit and mounds of grapes, fig trees all ripe with beautiful fruit (1)

We are beginning to move into our promised land, but the vineyards require work. "No tree requires such constant and severe pruning as the vine." (2) Taking care of vineyards requires a lot of care. God gave us instruction in Isaiah 5 for caring for a vineyard. It requires the land to be fertile. The soil has to be dug and cleared of stones, and the best vines are planted in the tended soil. Amid the vineyard are a watchtower, someone to keep watch and care for the vineyard, and last of all a wine vat for storage.

Isaiah 5 will be our guide for the week. We are ready to create a vineyard. The vineyard is our body, a place that you are actively working on these 40 days, building fertile soil, breaking things up to clear the stones, tending our branches, listening to our watchtower, and storing all the wisdom we gain on this journey.

Today's Tip: Let's Get Moving
One important factor in the healing process is getting those bones, muscles, ligaments, and tendon's moving again. If you've been moving all along, then it's time to set some new goals and move a little further. This week we will focus on this topic during "today's tip" with relatable research and practice to assist you with your goals. V. Gilbert Beers, author of *Finding Purpose in Your Pain*, said it best when he wrote, "Life at its best is an adventure. To live the adventure, you must risk getting hurt, for only through the adventure of living will you grow strong." What adventures are you currently planning? It's time to plan one.

Day 30:

Scripture Reading: Ezekiel 17: 1-10

Its branches turned toward him.
Ezekiel 17: 6a

Superior grapes are trained to grow upward. Often time farmers will begin their vineyards on hillsides to take advantage of this point. Planting a vineyard on a hill provides an ideal environment for fertile land; the right amount of heat, sunlight, water, and nutrients. (3)

We looked briefly at part of these verses before. God spoke through Ezekiel the prophet about a fallen king of Judah, the last king before the fall of Babylon. However, we can learn lessons from the parable about the vineyard we are planting. Ezekiel wrote, *"the seed started sprouting and the vine's branches begin to turn upward, and the roots stayed in place."* A second vine began to grow, it grew upward too, and its root was bent upward toward Him, so he could water it. This beautiful analogy is how we want to begin planting our vineyard, our new bodies where healing is its cornerstone. We need to always point our branches upward toward Him, so He can water our souls.

In this story, God was very angry at the Judean King. The king had sold out to another power, turned on his people, and later was destroyed. We need to heed God's warning about greed and turning our backs on Him. From the New Living Translation hear the words of the Lord.

So now the Sovereign Lord asks:
Will this vine grow and prosper?
No! I will pull it up, roots and all!
I will cut off its fruit

Nichole Fogleman

and let its leaves wither and die.
I will pull it up easily
without a strong arm or a large army.

But when the vine is transplanted,
will it thrive?
No, it will wither away
when the east wind blows against it.
It will die in the same good soil
where it had grown so well.

We do not want all of our hard work these forty days to be for nothing. The king in the story came from a good family. His story began as good, but he forgot to turn his branches upward and his vine forever withered away.

Today's Tip: Adventures Await
Get outside. My husband and I walk our dogs daily in a wildlife-permeated area. Early in the morning and in the evenings, we see deer, foxes, rabbits, osprey, snakes, and turtles. To view their habitat frequently throughout the year brings joy to our hearts. One morning recently, out of the blue I looked ahead and thought I saw a dinosaur. Mind you I did just see the latest Jurassic Park movie, but the dogs started running, my filters started processing, and for a brief moment I thought I saw a triceratops crossing the walkway. It was the largest most ancient-looking turtle I have ever seen, just minding his own business crossing the path, and after seeing us and two crazy dogs coming toward him, he became the fastest tortoise on record.

Getting out in nature never disappoints. Set up bird feeders and/or a birdhouse in your yard, if walking is out of the question right now in your journey. Take photos of the animals you see and share them with the ones you love. Your kids or significant may say they don't care, but they do. I love seeing photos my husband shares of his daily walk, even when it's a slithering snake.

Day 31:

Scripture Reading: Leviticus 25: 1-5

For six years you shall sow your field, and for six years you shall prune your vineyard and gather in its fruits,
but in the seventh year, there shall be a Sabbath of solemn rest for the land, a Sabbath to the Lord. Leviticus 25: 3-4

The work of a vineyard seems like it is never done, hoeing and breaking up the ground after the rain, pruning the vines, but even God rested on the seventh day while creating the earth. In our reading today from Leviticus, God emphasized the importance of resting the land in the 7th year. For one whole year, the Israelites had to rely completely on the provision of God, and the items they had stored. Even today in Israel to make kosher wine, the field must "lie fallow every 7th year." (3)

The question then comes up, are Christians required to follow the laws applied to the Sabbath? Some say Christ healed on the Sabbath, so this doesn't apply to me. God still is in the healing business. He heals 24/7 all over the world. He is in the business of healing our souls, even while we are sitting at church. But He is God. Charles Spurgeon stated "The Sabbath was a day of rest, and Christ did not break his rest by his miracles; for he was God, so it was rest to him to do good. (4)

I believe the body was designed to rest. When writing, I only write for six days at a time and then I rest. This study is designed for you to purposefully rest on the 7th day each week. We take this time to praise and worship the healing work God is doing in our bodies.

Sometimes it's difficult to rest. Let your loved ones know you will be doing this throughout these forty days. Depending on when you started this study, your day of rest may not fall on a Sunday or Saturday

In the Garden

and that's ok. You may be scheduled to work on those days. We are not going to be legalistic about it. Paul warned us in his letters about this.

The farmers had to plan to rest their fields in the 7th year. They were in the promised land now, there was no manna. They planned and stored food for survival. How are you going to spend your day of rejuvenation, refreshment, and revival? How are you going to plan your rest?

Plan it here.

_____

_____

_____

_____

_____

Today's Tip: Let's Get off That Couch
No matter what your fitness level is, the **Couch to Fitness** program led by Sport England is a great option. It's completely free and there are 3 levels of difficulty for each exercise with no equipment needed. There are multiple programs too including 30-minute workouts, smaller bitesize, five-minute workouts, Bhangra, and Aerobic dance sessions, and Family Fit sessions for the whole household. It's out of England, and professes to be free and always free, designed for beginners, three sessions per week.[iii]

[iii] https://couchtofitness.com/

Day 32:

Scripture Reading: Isaiah 5: 5-7

"We have to be broken to fee our life-giving gifts to those around us."
—Lynda Langhorne, former slave to chronic pain, diagnosis arachnoiditis

The best vines are planted in the tended soil. What type of soil is needed in a vineyard? So far in our vineyards, we have learned that the best fertile land is on a hill, looking upward; keeping our eyes set on our heavenly father. We have a plan for our vineyard, knowing we have to give it rest, and today we are going to talk about tending the soil; new growth emerging from brokenness.

To tend the soil, we have to break it. Hoe it. Break it into smaller and smaller pieces. These are special instruments used to break up the soil around vines. V. Gilbert Beers wrote in his book "Finding Purpose in Your pain," that productivity was directly related to the brokenness we inflicted on the soil. No farmer planted his crops without first breaking his soil as much as he could. (5) Brokenness is required to reap a harvest. How do those words feel? Do images of anger come to light as you think about how life at times can feel so broken? Record your thoughts below. Record a time recently when brokenness occurred in you or your family's life.

_____

_____

_____

In the Garden

I have mentioned before the quotes my mom underlined or wrote in the margins of books. Again and again, I am drawn to this book by Beers. In the chapter where Beers titled "Turn your Brokenness into Wholeness, Recreating the New You" my mom underlined these words "After a pot is broken and rebuilt, a pot has to be larger due to the glue that holds it together. We are a larger people when we are restored." Just like every spring when the vinedresser breaks the soil, He is hoping to create new life, to create whole beautiful grapes from the brokenness of the soil. Life may seem to be breaking apart but God can create wholeness in your life.

My mom, wrote at the peak of her pain; enduring gut-wrenching muscle spasms, incontinence of bowel and bladder, knife-sharp and day end and day out with no relief, "Me, I have entered brokenness, for my rebirth." Amen, mom. You went through hell and back, you lived in misery for 15 years, but you learned to tend your soil, rely on God, you planted your vineyard on a hill, and even in complete and utter brokenness, even in death, you are teaching us today.

The vineyard in our reading represented the nation of Israel, it had to be broken into a different way to experience life again. Hoeing and pruning were not enough. Their sins were so defiling that destruction, and trampling needed to occur. Let's heed this warning. Allow God to prune and hoe your soil.

Today's Tip: Yoga, it's not just for Yogi
There's promising evidence that yoga may help manage symptoms of those that suffer from chronic illness and improve their quality of life. Thus, yoga may be a helpful addition to your movement program. The National Center for Complementary and Integrative Health published an e-book in July 2022 addressing health and the practice of yoga. The following are recommendations and findings from this organization

regarding the use of yoga practice among patients that suffer from pain. Many other conditions are included in the e-book; asthma, MS, anxiety, diabetes, heart disease, and even COPD. Their website outlines 291 studies regarding yoga and chronic disease. In the reference area, there are three recent studies in case anyone wants to dig deeper. (7,8,9)

—Low-Back Pain. Studies of yoga for low-back pain have shown that it may reduce the intensity of the pain and help people function better, although the effect may be small. Based on this research, the American College of Physicians suggests yoga as one of several options for first-line nondrug treatment of chronic low-back pain. —

—Neck Pain. Only a small amount of research has been done on yoga for neck pain, but the results have been favorable. Yoga appears to have short-term benefits on both the intensity of neck pain and disability related to neck pain. —

—Headaches. Just a few studies have been done on yoga for headaches. However, only one rigorously conducted study has shown improvement. —

—Arthritis and Fibromyalgia. There hasn't been much research on yoga for osteoarthritis, rheumatoid arthritis, or fibromyalgia, but the small amount of research that's available suggests that yoga may be helpful for symptoms of these conditions. (6)

Day 33:

Scripture Reading: Psalm 127: 1-2, Psalm 61: 3, Matthew 21: 33, Habakkuk 2: 1-4

Unless the Lord watches over the city, the guards stand watch in vain.
Psalm 127: 1-2

In every vineyard in the Bible is a watchtower, placed to watch over the grapes and vines for intruders, pests, and wild animals. And in every village, watch towers were serving the same purpose for the people. Watchtowers were built to protect and provide refuge. They served as part of their defense system.

Do you have a plan of defense during challenging times? You name the challenge: temptation, mother-in-law visits, co-worker discrimination, an excruciating bout of back pain. Now is the time to create a defense system. Our key verse Psalm 122:1-2 written by King David, dedicated to his son, Solomon, knew an integral part of building a city, vineyard, or building. God is your watchtower. He is the integral source of protection from the enemy. *"The name of the Lord is a strong tower, the righteous man runs into it and is safe." Proverbs 18: 10*

Today spend some time creating a defense system. At the top of your list is "The name of the Lord. He is my Strong Tower."

"My Defense system" Exercise

Challenge: Anger at a loved one.
My plan:
1. I will call on the name of the Lord. He is my strong tower.
2. Quick prayer asking for help

3. Stay silent and walk away if possible
4. Have a distraction nearby, AirPods so I can listen to music to help my settle soul.

Ok. Your turn.

Challenge: _____

My defense in times of challenge.
1. I will call on the name of the Lord. He is my strong tower.

2._____

3._____

4._____

Today's Tip: The Right Yoga Program
The great thing about yoga is that it can be done in the comfort of your own home. No one has to see how inadequate your downward dog pose compares to your friends. Shut the door, find some carpet, roll up a blanket, check out a book from the library to practice different poses, or go to my favorite yogi, *Yoga with Adriene,* on YouTube. The great thing about *Yoga with Adriene* is that it is free and she does a 30-day practice at the beginning of each year. You don't have to wait for the new year to start, just subscribe to her YouTube channel and begin. She also has 10-minute yoga for beginners. I love her dog, Benji, he's a yoga regular.

Day 34:

Scripture Reading: Revelations 14: 17-20

"Take your sharp sickle and gather the clusters of grapes from the earth's vine, because its grapes are ripe." The angel swung his sickle on the earth, gathered its grapes, and threw them into the great winepress of God's wrath.
Revelations 14: 18b- 19

We finish this week with the last element in the vineyard, the winepress. The winepress is used to crush and trample the grapes, often with the winepress's feet. The images in our scripture are quite graphic in Revelations. Similar images are found in the book of Isaiah, all denoting God's wrath. It's easy to sugarcoat Christianity. Yes, we are called to love one another, but the reality of the concept of "fearing" the Lord is an essential element of the Christian journey.

Psalms 25: 14 states *"The secret of the Lord is with them that fear him, and he will show them his covenant"* Many verses depict the fear of the Lord as a key to understanding and obtaining wisdom. (Psalm 111:10, Proverbs 2:1-5, Proverbs 9:10, Proverbs 1:7) Solomon, author of Proverbs, when asked for any gift from God, he chose wisdom. The mysteries of God's word are great, and the more we study the more we understand. My wish for you and myself is to avoid God's wrath, avoid the figurative winepress of his anger. So I choose to listen to Solomon's instructions found in Proverbs 2. Rewrite these words below in your journal today.

My child, listen to what I say,
and treasure my commands.
Tune your ears to wisdom,

Nichole Fogleman

and concentrate on understanding.
Cry out for insight,
and ask for understanding.
Search for them as you would for silver;
seek them like hidden treasures.
Then you will understand what it means to fear the Lord,
and you will gain knowledge of God.
For the Lord grants wisdom!
From his mouth come knowledge and understanding.

Today's tip: Adventures Outside Your Neighborhood
After experiencing a bout of non-weight-bearing confinement and scooter mobility experience over a summer, I discovered a great new world of adventure: the national park passport program. The passport book costs $12.95, the cost of gas to drive to the destination, and the rest is free. The options are limitless. There are 491 national parks. Every state has options, the ranger stamps your passport, you get to see beautiful scenery you would never see, make new friends along the way, and capture memories you will never forget. Most of the sites are handicapped accessible. To find out more, go to *https://americasnationalparks.org/passport-to-your-national-parks/*

Day 35:

Your day of Rest

Nichole Fogleman

Recipe:
Flora's Pickled Okra

After my mother died, I found some treasured recipes from her mother; the grandmother that lived in the house on the lake. She daily ate fresh vegetables out of her garden. She would often freeze her vegetables, store them in a large freezer and pull them out when she was ready to cook. Okra was a centerpiece on the table at the H-LFT, often fried in oil. This is a recipe I found of hers using the technique of pickling the okra, which is far healthier. Adding garnishes to foods can create the zest you need to keep eating those vegetables. Okra has magnesium, Vitamins A, K C, and B6.

  1/2 cup salt
  4 cups white vinegar
  1 cup water
  MIX these and stir over low heat

  2 cloves garlic
  1 Tablespoon dill seed
  2 hot peppers
  okra
  MIX okra mixture

Pour hot liquid mixture over the okra mixture. Place in Jars. Let stand 21 days before opening. (*I'm not sure why 21 days is the magic number, but who am I to question a great southern cook from the 1960s*)

THE OLIVE TREE

For if you were cut from what is by nature a wild olive tree, and grafted, contrary to nature, into a cultivated olive tree, how much more will these, the natural branches, be grafted back into their own olive tree. Romans 11: 24

Day 36:

Scripture Reading: Genesis 8:6-12

And the dove came back to him in the evening, and behold, in her mouth was a freshly plucked olive leaf. Genesis 8:11

We come to our last tree of hope, the olive tree. Our reading today winds up our 40-day journey. Noah endured 40 days waiting for change. Every seven days he sent out a new bird to see if the waters had receded. And as the verse above says, the dove came back, and "behold, in her mouth was a freshly plucked olive leaf."

It's been almost 40 days in our journey, the waters are receding, and you are ready for this new life. Interestingly of all the trees in the world, the dove brought back an olive leaf. A tree to represent renewal, refreshment of our soul, and a new life.

For the past 40 days, I've shared bits and pieces of my story, my mom's life, and my family's legacy. The family legacy I refer to is my birth into a life with Christ. In the year 1978, my life changed for good and for bad. Jesus called a little girl forward to a new life, waving the olive branch to represent a victory for eternal life. She heard His voice. She ran without hesitation. But what she didn't know is that the inner beauty that created a new life in her that night was shining bright on the outside too.

Growing up in the 70s in the south equated with beauty pageants. Every school had one. Literally, in the same week, she walked down the aisle of her community church, and then she walked down the runway of a stage in a little school in the backwoods of Jefferson County Alabama. What judges of that pageant didn't know was that they saw **His** glow in her that night on the runway. The decision made at the beauty pageant that night changed her life forever.

At 8 years old, she couldn't comprehend the changes that were going to occur. It wasn't until 40 years later that she saw clearly what happened that night. Satan used the inner glow of God's beauty for his purposes. People say a little girl was changed by Christ and thought her outward beauty was the formula. She won the beauty pageant for the entire school. She was bombarded with favor and titillations. Her popularity soared from being unnoticed to tiaras and headlines in the local news. And with that newfound popularity, Satan planted his seeds of generational sin. What Satan did not plan on was the seeds that God planted were planted in fertile soil, already being cultivated by parents and grandparents that loved Him and were fighting for a new life for their family. Guess whose seeds won?

Everyone in that family began planting seeds in fertile soil, rewriting history, and passing on a legacy of new believers every year. I thank God for this story even though the testing part was extremely difficult and almost ruined my life but I'm here today to wave an olive branch of victory and to help you reach maturation much quicker than I ever did.

The olive tree can start bearing fruit within three years after being planted. We began this growing process of a healthier you, planting, cultivating, and pruning. My prayer is that with your healing taking place every day on the inside, your fruit begins to mature quickly, never forgetting the lessons learned on this journey.

Today's Tip: Advice from My Mom
Mom sent me an email in 2020 with the title "It's time to ditch the term chronic pain" and use the term "persistent pain". It's so hard being labeled with a chronic illness, especially if the illness is invisible. I've seen firsthand how people judged my mom. I've been with her in the hospital ER, seen her in unspeakable pain so much so that she couldn't even lay down in a car on the way there, we had to stop and pull over

so I could call an ambulance to place her on a stretcher. I watched as people rolled their eyes possibly thinking, "this one's crazy, she just wants drugs." Having an invisible illness is heart-wrenching. Every September is Invisible Illness month. **Honor those around you that may have "persistent pain."** They may have a smile on their face, but underneath they may be hurting from neuropathy from their diabetes, Lyme's disease from a tick bite, mental fogginess from covid long haulers syndrome, peripheral vascular disease of their feet, or _____ (you fill in the blank).

Day 37:

Scripture Reading: Romans 11: 17-24

But if some of the branches were broken off, and you, although a wild olive shoot, were grafted in among the others and now share in the nourishing root of the olive tree, do not be arrogant toward the branches.
Romans 11: 17- 18a

The olive tree, possibly dating back to the Garden of Eden, harvested in the winter, cured for months before it can be eaten, transverses the countryside of Israel, Italy, Spain, and Greece. The great thing about the wild olive tree, even the roots of a tree dating back to ancient times, if found, one can clean up around the plant, graft new plants onto the old roots and produce new species. This practice still takes place even today. (2) The roots survive for thousands of years.

Your roots are still here Father Abraham, however, since Christ's visit to earth the grafting process has changed. A whole new species was grafted to the root, the Gentile, the non-Jewish believer. We are truly blessed to be granted this privilege, granted heritage to this sacred root. But with privileges come temptations. Charles Spurgeon, *The Faithful Olive Tree*, stated "as olive trees, we shall never be out of the way of temptation as long as we are grown in the earthly gardens." (1)

Paul warns us in the book of Romans, our reading today, to be mindful of developing arrogance as new creatures in Christ. We need to be grateful for all God does for us, practicing gratitude daily. We must trust in God's kindness, and never stop trusting.

Let's reflect on gratitude today. As we venture forward into the promised land, eating and drinking the fruits of the vines and growing

In the Garden

ancient olives from roots dating back thousands of years, we cannot allow living in this great land to fill our heads with haughtiness.

One of the best practices I have developed over the years is the practice of gratitude. In the early 2000s, a multitude of research was done in the area of gratitude. Scientists found cardiac health benefits in the practice of gratitude: lowering blood pressure and lowering levels of stress. and depression. (3) I encourage you to begin a daily gratitude practice after we are done with this journey. There are many great books out there on this practice or just create your journal. A great accessory to acquire is Lara Casey's "Cultivate What Matter" journals. She created a Gratitude Journal from her "write the word" series. In each journal on each page is a different scripture to help guide your scripture study every day. (4) We have to armor ourselves when our 40 days are complete. Temptation most likely will increase because you found fertile soil. Be ready. Begin today.

King David wrote a treasured psalm of gratitude. Let's see how he did it.

Give thanks to the Lord, for he is good,
for his steadfast love endures forever.
Give thanks to the God of gods,
for his steadfast love endures forever.
Give thanks to the Lord of lords,
for his steadfast love endures forever;
to him who alone does great wonders,
for his steadfast love endures forever;
to him who by understanding made the heavens,
for his steadfast love endures forever;
to him who spread out the earth above the waters,
for his steadfast love endures forever;
to him who made the great lights,
for his steadfast love endures forever;
the sun to rule over the day,
for his steadfast love endures forever;

Nichole Fogleman

the moon and stars to rule over the night,
for his steadfast love endures forever;
Psalm 136: 1- 9

Now it's your turn. What are you grateful for today?

_____

_____

_____

_____

_____

_____

Today's Tip: More Practice with Gratitude
Make gratitude purposeful. I love Etsy; so many creative minds. I typed in "gratitude" in the search bar on Etsy searching for journals and there are 82,475 products made and sold about the practice of gratitude. People are beginning to understand the significance of this practice, but are they doing it? One idea I have found very helpful for me includes engaging in a social media gratitude practice for one month. This could be done at any time but do it for a specific cycle, 40 days would be a great number, and purposefully create "shoutouts" for all those things you are grateful for, and ultimately encourage others. I usually do this once a year and love the whole experience. I find myself searching earnestly for good content which makes the practice so much more fun.

Day 38:

Scripture Reading: Matthew 7:1-4, Romans 11: 23-24

And even they, if they do not continue in their unbelief, will be grafted in, for God has the power to graft them in again.
For if you were cut from what is by nature a wild olive tree, and grafted, contrary to nature, into a cultivated olive tree, how much more will these, the natural branches, be grafted back into their olive tree.
Romans 11:23-24

We continue to study the olive tree. Interestingly, olives cannot be eaten directly from the tree. They are very bitter. Olives must be cured to remove the bitterness. This practice of curing the olive takes many shapes and forms depending on the culture doing the curing. Originally, the first olives may have been soaked in salt water to cure them. (5)

Imagine we are grafted as individuals from the original olive tree to the tree of eternal life. We represent the olive, bitter without the Holy Spirit to make us more palatable. We are like the olive, requiring curing time to make us more like Christ. As we strive to be more like Christ, less judging of others, tempering our arrogance, and humbling our souls; let's be mindful that this is a process. Whether the olive is being cured gently by salt or rapidly by soaking it in lye. We can only hope the curing process for our souls occurs with a more gentle process.

From our scripture reading today, the olive tree reminds us of another lesson on avoiding temptation as we venture forth into the promised land. We are called to heed Christ's warning about the proclivity of judging others. If God can graft anyone back into the olive tree, who are we to judge and say who is not welcome into the body of Christ?

Over history, man has judged who is welcome to join the ranks of the Christian church. Adulterers were unwelcome. Unmarried and living in sin were unwelcome. The list goes on and on depending on the generation and the leader of the church.; you fill in the blank. God has His timing and works on the hearts of His creation. Jesus while dying on the cross invited a murderer to enter the thresholds of heaven at the same moment of his death. This was the monumental moment in history that the world had been waiting for since sin first entered the world with Adam and Eve. How astounding that He shared the limelight of his entrance back into Heaven with a murderer. Christ taught us that *"all of Heaven celebrates when the one sinner repents than over the 99 righteous people who no need to repent." (Luke 15:7) Christ said to this man "Truly I say to you, today you shall be with me in paradise." (Luke 23:42)*

Allow God to cure you. Cure you like the olive that must be forever changed to remove the bitterness. Allow God to transform you to be more like Christ; humble, not judging others, and concerned for our fellow brothers and sisters that are not believers, that they too will be grafted into their olive tree.

The pages of this book are devoted to those that suffer from chronic pain and illness. The invitation goes out to anyone, but you that suffer from relentless pain are the primary focus. Below I want you to place in writing your affliction that you would like to have "cured" by God. Rewrite the following very famous KJV verse about healing. Make it your own and lift your affliction in prayer to God today so that He may begin to cure you. His stripes from the cross were intended for your healing.

But he was wounded for our transgressions, he was bruised for our iniquities: the chastisement of our peace was upon him, and with his stripes, we are healed.
Isaiah 53:5

In the Garden

Today's Tip: Read Other's Testimonies of Healing
One of the most powerful books I ever read about healing was the story of Brian Wills in the book *10 Hours to Live: a True Story of Healing and Supernatural Living*. This book changed my life and how I view the power of healing post-resurrection of Christ. We read so many stories in the bible about Jesus physically healing individuals while He was here on earth, but does he still heal? I think that's a big fat "yes!!" Find motivation in their stories. I will forever be a believer in the power of healing because of his story.

Day 39:

Scripture Reading: Judges 9: 7- 21

…. If you really want to anoint me king over you, come and take refuge in my shade…
Judges 9: 15a

Generational sin is the culprit of so many devastating stories since man first walked this earth; stories of addiction, pain, suffering, and illness. The story I have intertwined about my own life in the ink of this book has been an attempt to hail victory and not pass down my own family's burdens. Today, we close on our next to the last day, a story taking place in the promised land, a man who followed God's lead, that had a tremendous victory for God, but then forgot to break the chain of sin and passed it on to his family with ultimate final destruction.

That man was Gideon. The parable from our scripture today, the parable about the olive tree, the fig tree, the vine, and the bramble, was written by Gideon's son Jotham. Gideon, a man born to a family that worshiped and idolized other gods, a man that was called by God to lead an army and fight an enemy, a man that humbly turned down a kingship after his victory, and a man that eventually forgot everything he learned along the way from defeat to victory. He created a symbol unknowingly for sin, and the symbol he created from the gold of his enemies, an ephod, (Judges 8: 27) eventually led a nation to fall.

Jotham, Gideon's son was trying to warn the people, and turn them away from the "bramble." The bramble was his brother. He saw that his father, the symbolic vine, forgot his covenant with God and passed along the burdens of his grandfather to his son. This son, evil in sight and deed, murdered all but one of his brothers and was eventually overthrown and killed.

What lessons are we to learn from this story? God is our King. There is no need for any other. "Make us like the nations around us," the Israelites cried. The olive from Jotham's parable spoke the most respectable reply of all "Am I no longer good for making oil?" The olive honored God by giving oil. Charles Spurgeon talked about the good olive in his sermon *The Faithful Olive Tree*, (1)" It was the olive's glory that it yielded oil which was used in various offerings to the honor of God ...And the highest glory of any man's life is that he is honorable to God and useful to men. The first consideration of a saved soul should be, "How can I best magnify Him who has saved me? How can I be most useful to my fellow men in promoting the cause of the Lord Jesus Christ?"

What are your talents? What are your gifts? How do you honor God? Just like the olive who gave oil to his kindred, we are all created with gifts to bestow, maybe it's crafting or maybe it's accounting for your sister's taxes.

_____

_____

_____

_____

_____

_____

Nichole Fogleman

Today's Tip: Join a Support Group

Since the covid epidemic, finding in-person support groups are few and far between. Finding others that have similar stories can be a very valuable tool for healing. These groups should not be a gripe session or a time to complain about doctors. Look for groups that mentor friendships, sharing, gratitude, and positive advice. There is a resource written by Lisa Copen, leader of Rest Ministries, called *How To Start A Chronic Illness Small Group Ministry*. We need more volunteers out there to lead these types of groups whether it's in person or by zoom. The U.S. Pain foundation does have support groups, but they still need more volunteers. They train their volunteers to lead these groups. According to their website, "they lead helpful techniques, like mediation, breathing exercises, guided images, decision-making models, role-playing, assertiveness skills." Two of their volunteers just published their books about chronic pain.[iv]

[iv] https://painconnection.org/support-groups/location-based-support-group-meetings/

Day 40:

Scripture Reading: Luke 22: 39-46, Acts 1: 1-12

Jesus went out as usual to the Mount of Olives, and his disciples followed him.
Luke 22:39

"Vineyards forsaken die out almost immediately, and fig orchards neglected run rapidly to ruin, but not so the olive," writes William Thomson author of the *Land and the Book*. (5) The value of the olive tree in ancient times was like no other, yielding invaluable wealth for the landowner. The fruit of this tree was used to nourish the body, give sight from its burning oil, and blessings from its production. The farmer "with no other provision than olives wrapped up in a bounty of his back, and with this, he was contented." (6) The olive tree is the tree in which all branches are grafted. The olive tree on our last day together will symbolize Jesus Christ. He is the ultimate producer of contentment. He provides all that we need, nourishment for our body, light for our soul, and blessings for our spirit.

Jesus's last days as a physical man on earth were among the olives. His ascension into heaven occurred among the olives at the Mount of Olives. (Acts 1: 1-12) After spending forty days with his disciples after his resurrection, he told them that a special gift would be coming from their Father. The Holy Spirit was that gift. (Acts 1:4) *"You will receive power when the Holy Spirit comes on you, and you will be my witnesses in Jerusalem, and in all Judea and Samaria, and to the ends of the earth."*

God has sewn a remarkable and undeniable thread through this bible study for you. We began in the fig orchard with Amos and pierced our souls to ripen our fruit, we descended to the fields to uncover the mystery of the seed, watered it with rains from the former and latter presence of God, we pruned the branches of the vine with the help of our heavenly savior, and ended in the olive grove with our savior's prayer and ascension. The thread ends today with you in the promised land and all the people of the world gathered for the harvest. The day the Holy Spirit ascended onto the multitude at Pentecost was *Shavuot,* the concluding harvest festival. The day that the harvest from the promised land fruit, the fig, the grape, the olive, (Deuteronomy 8:8) could be brought forward to give glory to God. We have finished the forty days. It's the day of the harvest.

And on that day of Pentecost, Peter spoke to the crowd, and he spoke the following, referencing the book of Joel

"I will pour out my Spirit on all people.
Your sons and daughters will prophesy,
your young men will see visions,
your old men will dream dreams.
Even on my servants, both men, and women,
I will pour out my Spirit in those days,
and they will prophesy.
I will show wonders in the heavens above
and signs on the earth below,
blood and fire and billows of smoke.
The sun will be turned to darkness
and the moon to blood
before the coming of the great and glorious day of the Lord.
And everyone who calls
on the name of the Lord will be saved.'
Joel 2:28-29

This is the ultimate message for all of us, the ones grafted to the original olive tree. Anyone who calls on him will be saved. He pours out his spirit. We, daughters and sons, are called to have a relationship

In the Garden

with Him, to prophecy is to speak, to hear the voice of the Lord. We all have this gift now. We on our journey the rest of these days on this earth, are called to have a relationship with Him. You undeniably can hear his voice. You only need to listen. Almost every single word throughout the Bible is about cultivating this relationship. We are not called as believers to exist until our earthly bodies deteriorate and then ascend to heaven. We are called to live, in the garden of life, alongside Him and to thrive.

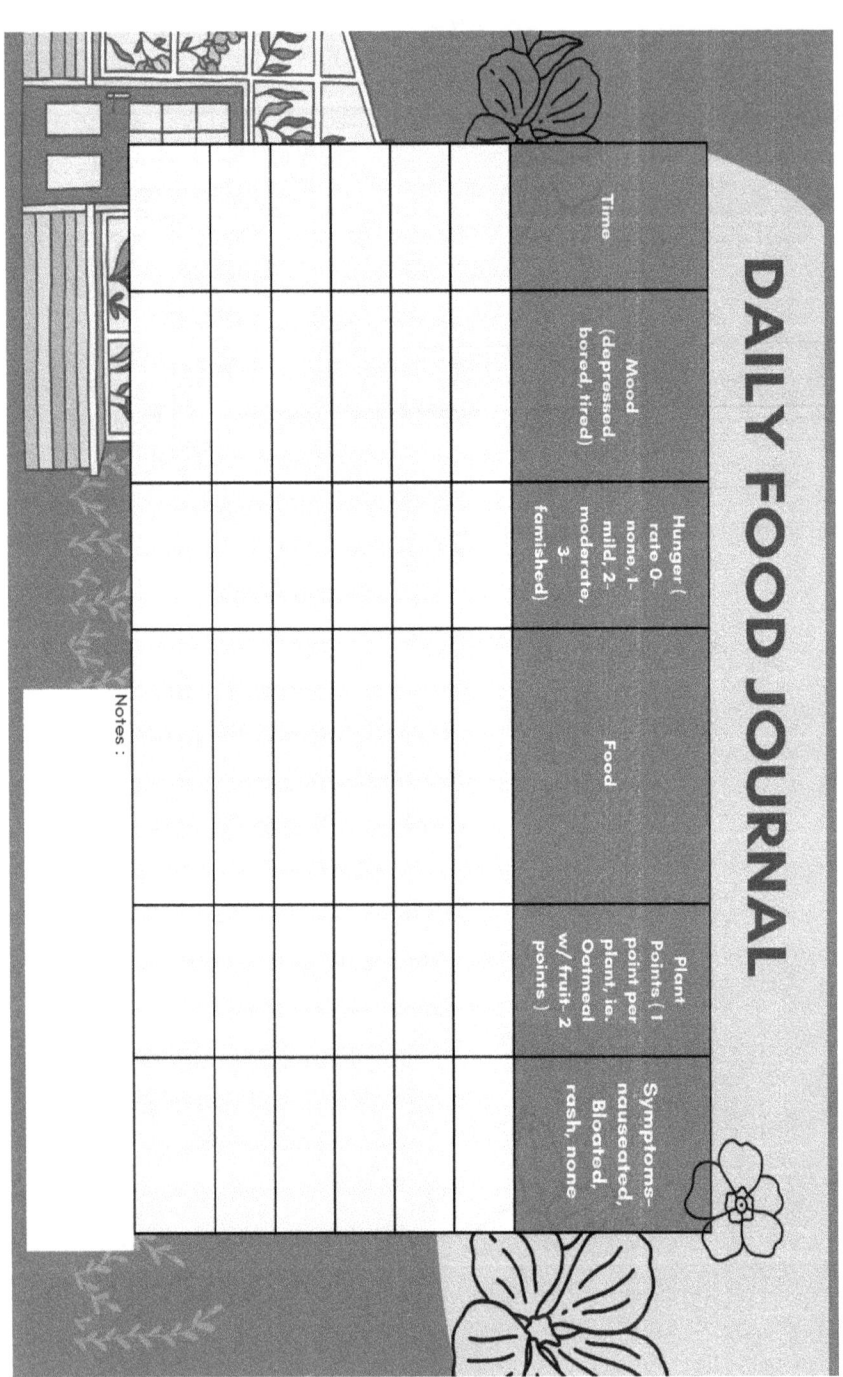

DAILY FOOD JOURNAL

Time	Mood (depressed, bored, tired)	Hunger (rate 0- none, 1- mild, 2- moderate, 3- famished)	Food	Plant Points (1 point per plant, ie. Oatmeal w/ fruit- 2 points)	Symptoms- nauseated, Bloated, rash, none

Notes :

About Kharis Publishing

Kharis Publishing, an imprint of Kharis Media LLC, is a leading Christian and inspirational book publisher based in Aurora, Chicago metropolitan area, Illinois. Kharis' dual mission is to give voice to under-represented writers (including women and first-time authors) and equip orphans in developing countries with literacy tools. That is why, for each book sold, the publisher channels some of the proceeds into providing books and computers for orphanages in developing countries so that these kids may learn to read, dream, and grow. For a limited time, Kharis Publishing is accepting unsolicited queries for nonfiction (Christian, self-help, memoirs, business, health and wellness) from qualified leaders, professionals, pastors, and ministers. Learn more at: About Us - Kharis Publishing - Accepting Manuscript

Cited reference

Chapter 1

1. Pollan, Michael. *Food Rules: An Eater's Manual.* New York: Penguin Books, 2009. Print.15, 41

2. Spurgeon, Charles. "Fellowship with Christ." *The Spurgeon Center*, 15 Jan. 1856, https://www.spurgeon.org/resource-library/sermons/fellowship-with-christ/#flipbook/

3. Malkmus, George H., et al. *The Hallelujah Diet: Experience the Optimal Health You Were Meant to Have.* Destiny Image Publishers, 2006.

4. *The Queen of Trees African Queen.* (n.d.). https://treesofjoy.com/wp-content/uploads/2017/03/NATURE-The-Queen-of-Trees-African-Queen-PBS.mp4.

5. Galil, J. An ancient technique for ripening sycamore fruit in East-Mediterranean Countries. *Econ Bot* **22**, 178–190 (1968). https://doi.org/10.1007/BF02860561

6. National Gardening Association survey, https://www.gardenresearch.com/index.php?q=show&id=3126

Chapter 2

1. Leichtle, S.W., Sarma, A.K., Strein, M. *et al.* High-Dose Intravenous Ascorbic Acid: Ready for Prime Time in Traumatic Brain Injury? *Neurocrit Care* 32, 333–339 (2020).

2. Barker, Tyler, et al. "Vitamin E and C supplementation does not ameliorate muscle dysfunction after anterior cruciate ligament surgery." *Free radical biology & medicine* vol. 47,11 (2009): 1611-8. doi: 10.1016/j.freeradbiomed.2009.09.0101. V. https://doi.org/10.1007/s12028-019-00829-x

3. Vanek VW, Borum P, Buchman A, et al. A.S.P.E.N. position paper: recommendations for changes in commercially available parenteral multivitamin and multi-trace element products. Nutr Clin Pract. 2012;27(4):440–91

4. Frei, B., Birlouez-Aragon, I., & Lykkesfeldt, J. (2012). Authors' Perspective: What is the Optimum Intake of Vitamin C in Humans? *Critical Reviews in Food Science and Nutrition, 52*, 815–829. https://doi.org/10.1080/10408398.2011.6491494.

5. Doseděl, Martin et al. "Vitamin C-Sources, Physiological Role, Kinetics, Deficiency, Use, Toxicity, and Determination." *Nutrients* vol. 13,2 615. 13 Feb. 2021, doi:10.3390/nu13020615

6. Padayatty, S., Katz, A., Wang, Y., Eck, P., Kwon, O., Lee, J.-H., Chen, S., Corpe, C., Dutta, A., Dutta, S., & Levine, M. (2003). Vitamin C as an Antioxidant: Evaluation of Its Role in Disease Prevention. *Journal of the American College of Nutrition, 22*, 18–35. https://doi.org/10.1080/07315724.2003.10719272

7. Beers, V. G. (1998). *Finding purpose in your pain*. F.H. Revell.

8. Barnard, N., & Raymond, J. (1998). *Food that fights pain: Revolutionary new strategies for maximum pain relief*. Harmony Books.

9. Bernstein AL. Vitamin B6 in clinical neurology. Annals of the New York Academy of Sciences. 1990; 585:250-260. DOI: 10.1111/j.1749-6632.1990.tb28058.x. PMID: 2162644.

10. Liz Curtis Higgs, *The Girl's Still Got it*, (Colorado Springs, WaterBrook Press, 2012), 107

11. Linda H. Hollies, *On Their Way too wonderful: A Journey with Naomi and Ruth* (Cleveland: Pilgrim Press, 2004), 24.

12. Herrmann, W., & Geisel, J. (2002). Vegetarian lifestyle and monitoring of vitamin B-12 status. In *Clinica Chimica Acta* (Vol. 326, Issues 1–2). https://doi.org/10.1016/S0009-8981(02)00307-8

13. Scott, J. M. "Bioavailability of vitamin B12." *European journal of clinical nutrition. Supplement* 51.1 (1997): S49-S53.

14. Del Bo', C., Riso, P., Gardana, C., Brusamolino, A., Battezzati, A., & Ciappellano, S. (2019). Effect of two different sublingual dosages of

vitamin B12 on Cobalamin nutritional status in vegans and vegetarians with a marginal deficiency: A randomized controlled trial. *Clinical Nutrition*, *38*(2), 575–583. https://doi.org/10.1016/j.clnu.2018.02.008

15. https://hebrewwordlessons.com/2019/08/04/zera-a-seed-in-the-garden/

16. Urits, Ivan et al. "Utilization of Magnesium for the Treatment of Chronic Pain." *Anesthesiology and pain medicine* vol. 11,1 e112348. 6 Feb. 2021, doi:10.5812/aapm.112348

17. Pennington, J. A. T., *Bowes and Chruch's Food Values of Portions Commonly Used*, 16th ed. (Philadelphia: J. B. Lippincott, 1994).

18. Swanson, Don R. "Migraine and Magnesium: Eleven Neglected Connections." *Perspectives in Biology and Medicine*, vol. 31 no. 4, 1988, p. 526-557. *Project MUSE*, doi:10.1353/pbm.1988.0009.

19. Morgan, Robert. *Reclaiming the Lost Art of Biblical Meditation: Find True Peace in Jesus*. Vida, 2021.

20. Spurgeon, Charles, The Complete Works of Charles Spurgeon, Volume 46: Sermons 2603-2655, Delmarva Publications, Inc.,

21. Chakraborty AJ, Mitra S, Tallei TE, Tareq AM, Nainu F, Cicia D, Dhama K, Emran TB, Simal-Gandara J, Capasso R. Bromelain a Potential Bioactive Compound: A Comprehensive Overview from a Pharmacological Perspective. *Life*. 2021; 11(4):317. https://doi.org/10.3390/life11040317

22. Jurek, Scott. *Eat and Run: My Unlikely Journey to Ultramarathon Greatness*. Mariner Books, 2013.

23. BULSIEWICZ, W. I. L. L. (2022). *Fiber fueled: The plant-based gut health program for losing weight, restoring your health, and... optimizing your microbiome.* AVERY PUB GROUP. p. 82

24. Panahi, Yunes, et al. "Effects of curcumin on serum cytokine concentrations in subjects with metabolic syndrome: A post-hoc analysis of a randomized controlled trial." *Biomedicine & pharmacotherapy = Biomedicine & pharmacotherapy* vol. 82 (2016): 578-82. doi:10.1016/j.biopha.2016.05.037

In the Garden

25. Sahoo, J. P., Behera, L., Praveena, J., Sawant, S., Mishra, A., Sharma, S. S., Ghosh, L., Mishra, A. P., Sahoo, A. R., Pradhan, P., Sahu, S., Moharana, A., & Samal, K. C. (2021). *The Golden Spice Turmeric (Curcuma Longa) and its feasible benefits in prospering human health—a review. American Journal of Plant Sciences,* 12(03), 455–475. https://doi.org/10.4236/ajps.2021.123030

Chapter 3

1. BULSIEWICZ, W. I. L. L. (2022). *Fiber fueled: The plant-based gut health program for losing weight, restoring your health, and... optimizing your microbiome.* AVERY PUB GROUP.

2. Davis, E. F., & Berry, W. (2014). *Scripture, culture, and agriculture: An agrarian reading of the Bible.* Cambridge University Press.

3. Moore, Beth, *When Godly People Do Ungodly Things,* (Nashville, Broadman and Holman Publishers, 2002), all of chapter 3. , p. 34

4. Strong, James. *Strong's Exhaustive Concordance of the Bible.* Abingdon Press, 1890. Print.

5. Kosīte, D., König, L.M., De-loyde, K. *et al.* Plate size, and food consumption: a pre-registered experimental study in a general population sample. *Int J Behav Nutr Phys Act* **16,** 75 (2019). https://doi.org/10.1186/s12966-019-0826-1

5. Kosīte, D., König, L.M., De-loyde, K. *et al.* Plate size and food consumption: a pre-registered experimental study in a general population sample. *Int J Behav Nutr Phys Act* **16,** 75 (2019). https://doi.org/10.1186/s12966-019-0826-1

6. Korkiakoski A, Niinimäki J, Karppinen J, et al. Association of lumbar arterial stenosis with low back symptoms: a cross-sectional study using two-dimensional time-of-flight magnetic resonance angiography. *Acta Radiol.* 2009;50(1):48-54. doi:10.1080/02841850802587862

7. Peter C Coyle, PT, DPT, PhD, Victoria A O'Brien, PhD, David G Edwards, PhD, Ryan T Pohlig, PhD, Gregory E Hicks, PT, PhD, FAPTA, Markers of Cardiovascular Health in Older Adults with and Without Chronic Low Back and Radicular Leg Pain: A Comparative

Analysis, *Pain Medicine*, Volume 22, Issue 6, June 2021, Pages 1353–1359, https://doi.org/10.1093/pm/pnaa426

8. Barnard, N., & Raymond, J. (1998). *Food that fights pain: Revolutionary new strategies for maximum pain relief.* Harmony Books. p. 11

9. Esselstyn, C. B. (2011). *Prevent and reverse heart disease: The revolutionary, scientifically proven, nutrition-based cure.* Avery.

10. Esselstyn CB Jr, Ellis SG, Medendorp SV, Crowe TD. A strategy to arrest and reverse coronary artery disease: a 5-year longitudinal study of a single physician's practice. *J Fam Pract.* 1995;41(6):560-568.

11. Spurgeon, C. H. (Charles Haddon), 1834-1892. Sermons Du Rev. C. H. Spurgeon (New York: Sheldon, Blakeman, and Co, 1869), https://www.spurgeon.org/resource-library/sermons/the-former-and-the-latter-rain/#flipbook/

Chapter 4

1. Evans, Sydney, et al. "Cumulative risk analysis of carcinogenic contaminants in the United States drinking water." *Heliyon* vol. 5,9 e02314. 19 Sep. 2019, doi:10.1016/j.heliyon.2019.e02314

2. David Q. Andrews, and Olga V. Naidenko. "Population-wide Exposure to Per- and Polyfluoroalkyl Substances From Drinking Water In the United States." *Environmental science & technology letters*, v. 7,.12 pp. 931-936. doi: 10.1021/acs.estlett.0c00713

3. Javidi, A., & Pierce, G. (2018). U.S. Households' Perception of Drinking Water as Unsafe and Its Consequences: Examining Alternative Choices to the Tap. *Water Resources Research, 54.* https://doi.org/10.1029/2017WR022186

4. Mazur, M et al. "Oral health in a cohort of individuals on a plant-based diet: a pilot study." *La Clinica terapeutica* vol. 171,2 (2020): e142-e148. doi:10.7417/CT.2020.2204

5. Nave, Orville, J. "Nave's Topical Bible, A Digest of the Holy Scriptures," The Abingdon Press, New York 1896.

6. Hakim, M., Kurniani, N., Pinzon, R., Tugasworo, D., Basuki, M., Haddani, H., Pambudi, P., Fithrie, A., & Wuysang, A. (2018). Management of peripheral neuropathy symptoms with a fixed dose combination of high-dose vitamin B1, B6, and B12: A 12-week prospective non-interventional study in Indonesia. *Asian Journal of Medical Sciences*, *9*(1), 32-40. https://doi.org/10.3126/ajms.v9i1.18510

7. Calderón-Ospina CA, Nava-Mesa MO. B Vitamins in the nervous system: Current knowledge of the biochemical modes of action and synergies of thiamine, pyridoxine, and cobalamin. CNS Neurosci Ther. 2020 Jan;26(1):5-13. doi: 10.1111/cns.13207. Epub 2019 Sep 6. PMID: 31490017; PMCID: PMC6930825.

8. Héctor A. Ponce-Monter, Mario I. Ortiz, Alexis F. Garza-Hernández, Raúl Monroy-Maya, Marisela Soto-Ríos, Lourdes Carrillo-Alarcón, Gerardo Reyes-García, Eduardo Fernández-Martínez, "Effect of Diclofenac with B Vitamins on the Treatment of Acute Pain Originated by Lower-Limb Fracture and Surgery," *Pain Research and Treatment*, vol. 2012, Article ID 104782, 5 pages, 2012. https://doi.org/10.1155/2012/104782

Chapter 5

1. Trumbull, Henry Clay, *Kadesh-Barnea, Studies of the Route of the Exodus and the southern boundary of the Holy Land, (New York, Charles Scribner S Sons, 1884)*

2. Tristram, Henry Baker. 1868 *The Natural History of the Bible: being a review of the physical geography, geology, and meteorology of the Holy Land, with a description of every animal and plant mentioned in Holy Scripture.* 2nd ed. London: Society for Promoting Christian Knowledge., p. 408

3. Rogov, Daniel *The Ultimate Rogov's Guide to Israeli Wines, (New Milford, The Toby Press, 2012), 184*

4. Spurgeon, Charles. "Sabbath-Work." *The Spurgeon Center*, 18 Feb. 1883, https://www.spurgeon.org/resource-library/sermons/sabbath-work/#flipbook/.

5. Beers, V. G. (1998). *Finding purpose in your pain.* F.H. Revell.

6. https://files.nccih.nih.gov/s3fs-public/Yoga-eBook-2020_06_FINAL_508.pdf, chapter 11

7. Long C, Ye J, Chen M, Gao D, Huang Q. Effectiveness of yoga therapy for migraine treatment: A meta-analysis of randomized controlled studies. Am J Emerg Med. 2022 Aug;58:95-99? doi: 10.1016/j.ajem.2022.04.050. Epub 2022 May 2. PMID: 35660369.

8. Anheyer D, Haller H, Lauche R, Dobos G, Cramer H. Yoga for treating low back pain: a systematic review and meta-analysis. Pain. 2022 Apr 1;163(4):e504-e517.

9. Denham-Jones L, Gaskell L, Spence N, Tim Pigott. A systematic review of the effectiveness of yoga on pain, physical function, and quality of life in older adults with chronic musculoskeletal conditions. Musculoskeletal Care. 2022 Mar;20(1):47-73.

Chapter 6

1. Spurgeon, C. H. (1879, May 29). *The Faithful Olive Tree.*, Spurgeon's Sermon Notes. N.p., Kregel Publications, 1990., p. 29

2. Rosenblum, M., Olives the Life and Lore of a Noble Fruit, (New York, North Point Press, 1996) pp. 10,13,32

3. McCraty, Rollin, and Doc Childre. "12 The Grateful Heart The Psychophysiology of Appreciation." *The psychology of gratitude* 230 (2004).

4. Casey, L. Cultivate: A Grace-Filled Guide to Growing an Intentional Life, Write the Word journal, website: www.cultivatewhatmatters.com

4. Maier, Paul; *In the Fullness of Time: A Historian Looks at Christmas, Easter, and the Early Chruch*, United States, Kregel Publications, 1991, 130, 135

5. Thomson, William McClure. The Land and the Book: Or, Biblical Illustrations Drawn from the Manners and Customs, the Scenes, and Scenery of the Holy Land. United Kingdom, Harper, 1859., p. 73, 78

www.ingramcontent.com/pod-product-compliance
Lightning Source LLC
Chambersburg PA
CBHW070159100426
42743CB00013B/2980